Still
in My Arms

a devotional about a Mothers healing after
the stillbirth of her daughter

Amy E. von Oven

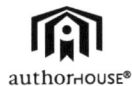

authorHOUSE®

AuthorHouse™
1663 Liberty Drive
Bloomington, IN 47403
www.authorhouse.com
Phone: 1-800-839-8640

First published by AuthorHouse   06/02/2011

ISBN: 978-1-4567-4864-7 (ebk)
ISBN: 978-1-4567-4865-4 (hc)
ISBN: 978-1-4567-4866-1 (sc)

Library of Congress Control Number: 2011908615

Printed in the United States of America

Any people depicted in stock imagery provided by Thinkstock are models, and such images are being used for illustrative purposes only. Certain stock imagery © Thinkstock.

Dedicated to our Sweet Daughter

Bethany Hope von Oven

May 3, 2009
7 lbs 3oz 21 in
Forever in our hearts

About Me

I am a thirty year old wife and mother of four children. My husband Brad and I have been married for ten years and he has been my rock throughout this battle in our lives. This journey has truly changed us forever as we are learning to live life again with our children.

I just recently completed my Bachelor's Degree in Early Childhood Education, although I have been blessed to be a stay at home mom for the last ten years. We live in Georgia with our children who are eleven, eight and five. Each and every day they teach me that life is a blessing and they are a miracle. I have learned that life is short and to never take any moment for granted. God is the giver of life, and we are not guaranteed our next breath. Today and everyday, God allows me to remain on this Earth and I choose to live for Him and glorify His name.

Table of Contents

Day 1- The beginning

"Blessed are those who mourn, for they will be comforted."
Matthew 5:4

May 3, 2009 is a day I will never forget. Although many of the memories are vague in my mind, I will never forget the reality of that day! May 2, was a beautiful Saturday filled with joy and laughter. I woke up anxious and exited to start the day. I was having a baby shower at our church, and although I am always nervous at social gatherings with me as the center of attention, I was elated.

The baby shower was beautiful and yet exhausting. By the time I returned home I had been gone a total of five hours. I was tired, swollen, hungry, and all of the other so called clichés very pregnant women seem to experience late in pregnancy!

It had been a long hot day, not to mention that I was 37 weeks pregnant and feeling rather large and ready for this baby to come. I quietly sat in the nursery and put away the wonderful gifts we had received and laughed at all the pink stuff we had been given, considering we did not know if it was a boy or girl!

Later that evening I finally crawled into bed to crash for the night. I gently placed my hands on my stomach expecting the baby to be moving, as she had done every night prior to this. As I anxiously watched the time continue to tick by with still no movement, I began to worry. My husband started pushing on my stomach and there was still no movement. After an hour, I decided I needed to head to the doctor.

I can still remember praying all the way to hospital that everything would be ok, but I think I knew that it was not ok. When I got to the hospital they quickly got me into a room and tried to find the baby's heartbeat and yet a chilling silence saturated the entire room. I was beginning to feel very sick as they rolled the ultrasound machine over my stomach to reveal a curled up and lifeless baby girl. I laid my head back and cried, "God no, God why?"

The next few hours are somewhat of a blur. I don't think I talked much; I just laid and cried. The next morning was Sunday, May 3, 2009. I was in a delivery room being induced to deliver my stillborn little girl. While most of the day is lost in my memories, I do remember the moment she was born. Three pushes and out she came. I did not see her - I simply laid my head back and closed my eyes as tears rolled down my face. My husband watched as her lifeless body came into the world. He fell to his knees and sobbed as he tightly held my hand.

Father, my whole body is numb as I fall into your arms. This moment in my life feels as though I have fallen into a dark hole. Hold me tight and guide me as I find my way through the unknown. Amen.

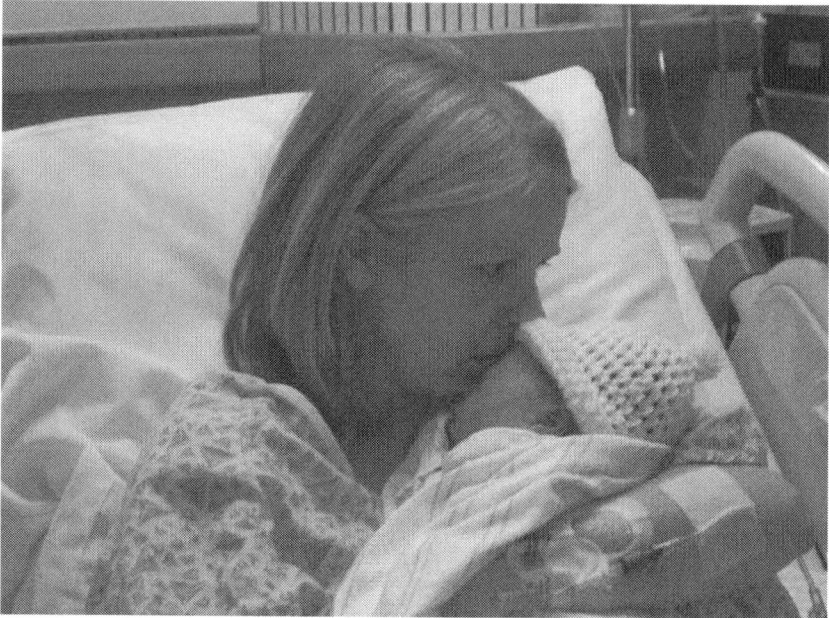

~I remember shaking uncontrollably as I sat in the cold hospital room waiting for my doctor to come in. I so desperately wanted my baby to start moving and for this to all be a very bad mistake. I could feel the presence of God so deeply, as if He was telling me that there was no mistake; she was really gone. What moments do you recall from your baby's birth?

Day 2-The Hospital

"My God, my God, why have You forsaken me?
Why are You so far from saving me, from the words of my
groaning?
O my God, I cry by day, but You do not answer,
and by night, but I find no rest" Psalms 22: 1-2

I was coming to as the drugs they had given me had begun to wear off, and I see what appears to be a shadow walking toward me with a blanket in her arms. Tears begin to flow from my eyes as she places my little girl into my arms.

I gently pull her close and sweetly kiss her head as I look at how perfect she appears. I can feel the silence in the room and see the tears falling from all who surround me, and yet I feel as though this can't be real. I lay Bethany on the bed gently cradling her head and began to dress her and carefully examine her perfect little body. I run my hand through her thick wavy black hair and lift her eyelid to see her blue eyes. She was truly perfect and breathtaking.

My heart is pleading for her to open her eyes and this all be a mistake and yet she sweetly lays there, no motion, no sound...she's really gone! My motherly instincts cannot accept that she is gone and I begin to worry because her skin is cold. I wrapped the blanket tightly around her, as I had always done with my other children, and I begin to wonder how I tell my children that their sister is not coming home.

I felt so still and lost.

I held her tiny face next to mine as I softly cried in disbelief. Brad crawled in the bed beside me as we both stared at her. I remember thinking, "Now what?" I had pictured this moment in my head a million

5

times: dressing her, nursing her, and simply enjoying the quiet time in the hospital before we went home to joyous noise and confusion. Never once did I picture myself holding my lifeless daughter who was already in the arms of Jesus.

I whispered in her ear that I loved her and she was in great hands, although my heart sunk to my stomach as I said these words. My mind was empty as I rolled over and cuddled her in my arms. I drifted off to sleep with her tightly beside me; I'm not sure anyone could have pried her from my arms at this point. I woke up and saw her sweet face and for a split second prayed she was breathing. Her chilling face and red lips quickly reminded me that she was not.

We knew it was time to let go, but how do you say goodbye to a life you have safely held under your heart for 9 months? And now I was just supposed to hand her over?

I grasped her tightly against my body as I once again whispered through the tears how much I loved her and already missed her. As I handed her over to the nurse my body collapsed into Brad's arms as we sobbed together.

My life was forever changed, and this room was forever part of those memories...I would never be the same!

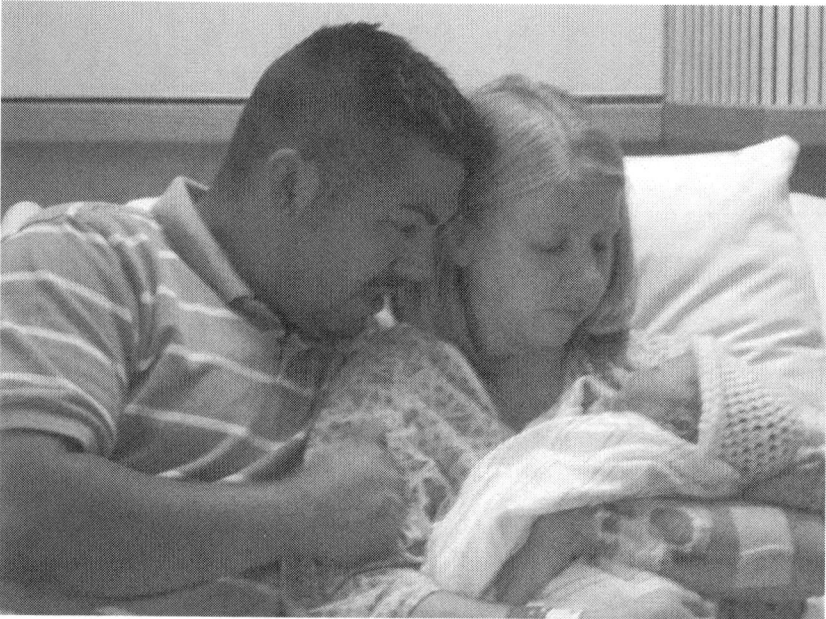

~Follow your heart in telling other children about the death of a sibling. We felt God telling us it would be too much on them to see her blue body and bright red lips. There is no right or wrong. God will lead your heart. Do not second guess yourself with whatever decision you make. Know that God is leading you and will continue to lead you. Where is your heart today?

Day 3-May 6-The Memorial Lunch

"The LORD is my rock, my fortress and my deliverer; my God is my rock, in whom I take refuge. He is my shield and the horn of my salvation, my stronghold."

Psalm 18:2

I step out of bed this morning feeling as though my body is standing still in time. My heart is beating so quickly and my face is swollen from tears.

I fall to the floor in my bathroom and bury my head in a towel as the tears again begin to uncontrollably flow from my eyes. I have no desire to do anything other than waste away in the covers of my bed and yet I can't. I have to get dressed and go to my daughter's funeral.

I cry out for God to take this pain away, to change something, anything to make this moment in my life be different. I'm reminded of Jesus praying in the garden before His crucifixion. How He cried out for His Father to take this cup from Him, but ultimately He knew it was God's will for Him to die on the cross.

I somehow manage to get off the floor and pull myself together, although my eyes are so blurry I can barely see to get dressed. I believe God is whispering in my ear, "Be still, I have a plan". My mind cannot grasp the concept of God's plan in taking my little girl from me, but I'm also reminded that God will walk me through this moment in my life if I just take His hand.

I managed to get dressed and I walked into my kitchen to take whatever pain medicine I could find to get me through this day. The car ride that morning was like a cartoon where the deepest darkest cloud simply stayed over our car as we drove.

We had a memorial lunch at our church that morning before the funeral. We pulled into the funeral home on our way to church for Brad to drop off a beautiful canvas picture of Bethany Hope. I watched as my husband carried our daughter's picture in and then walked out with tears rolling down his face. I watched him as he gently grabbed my hand and drove to the church with a silence I had never seen from him before. The last few days he had seemed so strong, or was I too hurt to notice his pain that I could so evidently see on his face this morning?

As we arrived at the church I could not get out of the car. I sat and cried. How do I see people or talk to people that just days before I had talked to about the excitement of having a baby any day?

I finally walked hand and hand with Brad into the church where our parents and church family waited to greet us with loving arms. I cried as they each hugged me as if it was someone else they were hugging. I was distant and not really there. I sat staring at a plate of food in front of me, not wanting to eat or say anything. I could barley focus on the talk coming from the people at my table and even laughter coming from my children.

I did not belong and I so desperately wanted to wake up from this never ending nightmare I was so deeply embedded in.

My husband then stood to read the words of a song God had lead him to find the night before. He changed a few of the words and again my eyes filled with tears as the words revealed what my heart was feeling:

Hello God, it's me again. 2:00 a.m., Room 304.
Visiting hours are over, time for our bedside tug of war.
This sleeping child between us may not make it through the night.
I'm fighting back the tears as she fights for her life.
Well, it must be kind of crowded,
On the streets of Heaven.
So tell me: what do you need her for?
Don't you know one day she'll be your little girl forever?
But right now I need her so much more.
She's much too young to be on her own:
Barely even born.
So who will hold her hand when she crosses the streets of Heaven?
She'll want to ride a pony when she's big enough.
She'll want to marry her Daddy when she's all grown up.
Lord, she is my angel
You've got plenty of your own
And I know you hold a place for her
But she's already got a home
Well Lord I know you're listenin'
So praying's all that's left to do
So I ask you Lord have mercy, you lost a Son once too
And it must be kind of crowded,
On the streets of Heaven.
So tell me: what do you need her for?
Don't you know one day she'll be your little girl forever?
But right now I need her so much more.
Lord, I know you've made your mind up
and there is no use in beggin'.
So when you take her with you today,
will you make sure she looks both ways,
And would you hold her hand when she crosses the streets of Heaven.

~Finding God's plan in the midst of death can seem confusing and feel overwhelming. It can be hard to search for any ray of light at the end of a tunnel when the tunnel is blocked by darkness. Open your heart to God and allow Him to slowly take away the darkness in your life. Allow yourself time to feel, hurt and cry, all while in the arms of Jesus. Where is your heart today?

Day 4-The Funeral

"The LORD is my shepherd, I shall not be in want. He makes me lie down in green pastures, He leads me beside quiet waters, He restores my soul. He guides me in paths of righteousness for His name's sake. Even though I walk through the valley of the shadow of death, I will fear no evil, for You are with me; Your rod and Your staff, they comfort me. You prepare a table before me in the presence of my enemies. You anoint my head with oil; my cup overflows. Surely goodness and love will follow me all the days of my life, and I will dwell in the house of the LORD forever." Psalm 23

My heart was pounding as we pulled into the parking lot of the funeral home. I remember looking around thinking that this place would forever be part of my life and my memories.

I walked inside the entry way and stared at the doors leading into my daughter's funeral. What I'm sure was only a few seconds seemed like an eternity as they started to open the doors.

I took about three steps and then there it was. I did not see the canvas picture or beautiful flowers surrounding her; I simply saw the smallest little urn sitting on this small round table and my heart sunk and my knees buckled. I was not sure I could keep going.

I remember sitting at the table the day before as they brought in the urns for me to see. I'm not sure what I had pictured, but I was in shock at how tiny they were. Just the thought of my daughter being in this tiny little vase that could fit into the palm of my hand made me nauseous and sick. They asked me to pick one out like I was picking a dish at a restaurant. Piece of cake, RIGHT?

One of our pastors quickly assured me that we could find something perfect to fit the urn inside of. We came to the decision to cremate Bethany because we are not sure if we will live in Georgia permanently and I would never leave Bethany behind if we buried her. Our pastor suggested that if we had her cremated, she could be buried in my casket with me one day.

Seeing the urn as I walked to the front of the church was a reminder that Bethany was gone and all that was left were her tiny remains in this tiny little vase, "How do I keep moving?"

Somehow I made it to the front of the church and sat down as I sobbed on my husband's shoulder.

Why was this hard?

I could never have prepared myself for something like this and yet here I was with a front seat view to my own daughter's funeral. It just doesn't seem right. I listened as our pastor began to talk and the tears began to flow even more. I was touched by his words. I was honored at how perfectly he spoke of her name, Bethany Hope, and the biblical meanings behind such a breathtaking name. I listened as a friend sang the words to one of my favorite songs, "You Are My All in All".

I remember thanking God at that moment for carrying me through this and being my all when I had nothing left of myself. We left the funereal and I came home and crawled into bed. I had somehow spaced out the people and voices circulating throughout my home and slipped away into the covers. I think part of me just wanted that day to be over. I drifted off to sleep as I sang the following words through the tears hitting my pillow:

<u>Words to You Are My All and All</u>
You are my strength when I am weak
You are the treasure that I seek
You are my all in all
Seeking You as a precious jewel
Lord to give up, I'd be a fool
You are my all in all
Jesus, Lamb of God, worthy is Your name
Jesus, Lamb of God, worthy is Your name
Taking my sin, my cross, my shame
Rising again, I bless Your name
You are my all in all
When I fall down, You pick me up
When I am dry, You fill my cup
You are my all in all

"Thank you, Father, for being my all when I am so empty and lost. Thank you for loving me and picking me up when grief and pain seem to seep into my soul and take over. Thank you for being stronger than all of my insecurities. Thank you for loving me. Amen.

For this is God, Our God forever and ever; He will be our guide
even to death. Psalms 48:14

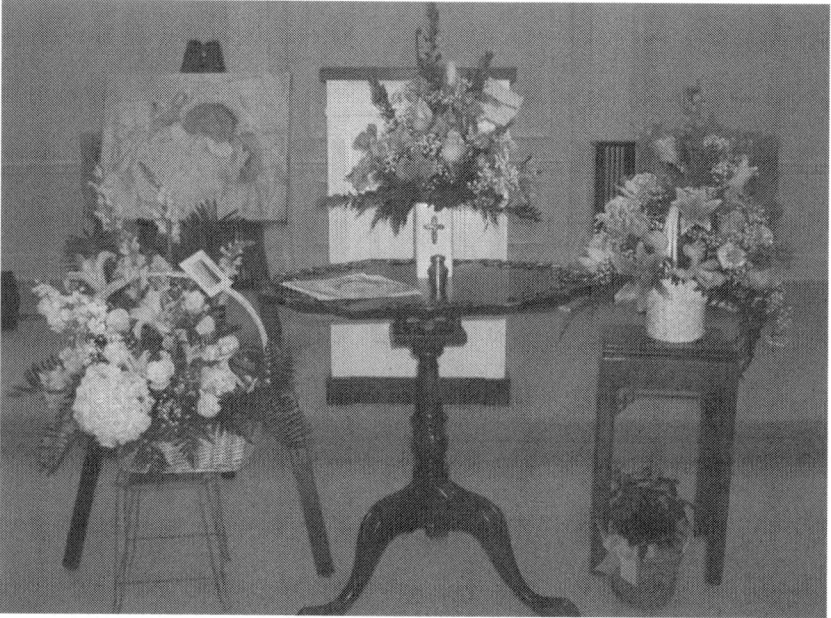

~Attending your own child's funeral is one of the hardest things a parent can do. Your heart might be numb right now and your body might simply being going through the motions; that's ok. Write about your child's funeral here or write about how you are feeling today.

_____

_____

_____

_____

_____

_____

_____

_____

_____

_____

_____

_____

_____

_____

_____

_____

_____

_____

_____

_____

_____

_____

_____

_____

_____

_____

_____

_____

_____

_____

_____

_____

_____

_____

Day 5- Prayers

"Do not be anxious about anything, but in everything,
by prayer and petition, with thanksgiving, present your
requests to God. And the peace of God, which transcends all
understanding, will guard your hearts and your minds in Christ
Jesus." Philippians 4:6-7

What happens when your answered prayers turn into, "What went wrong?" After the birth of our third child, Brayson Michael, Brad and I were transferred to New York with his job. We were scared and completely broke as a family of five.

Out of complete fear and anxiety, we choose for Brad to get a vasectomy. Two years later we were living in New Mexico and no longer worried about our finances and started to realize that we had made a mistake.

I first started to spend a lot of time in prayer trying to figure out what God's plan for us must be. I was scared and worried that Brad would never go through a reversal to have a fourth child, but soon realized that God had been working on his heart. He spoke to me on a car drive one day and said that he wanted to have the reversal done.

WHAT?

My heart was pounding! I could not believe this was even coming out of his mouth, I mean I could not believe he was really willing to go through that pain not once but twice, and for me! My dream and desire to add a fourth child might just come true, I was estactic!

As we began to look for a doctor, I slowly started to become discouraged because they were all charging way more money then we could ever spend. I again continued to pray for God's will and guidance knowing that we had exactly $1, 500 set aside to pay for the reversal. A few weeks later Brad called me from work to tell me that he had not only found a doctor, but found a Christian doctor who only charged a small flat fee of, get this, $1,500. I remember hanging up the phone and jumping up and down like a little kid who just got their favorite toy, I was thrilled!

Exactly 4 months after Brad's reversal I woke one morning starving, as if I had never had food before in my life. Of course my mind wondered if maybe there was more to this hunger, so I quickly ran to the bathroom and grabbed one of the many pregnancy tests I seemed to have stock in and could not believe what it revealed.

I was not sure if I should smile, cry, or stare at the test in complete amazement wondering if I was simply imagining two lines there (like I'm the only one who has ever done this).

My overwhelming joy was quickly shattered a long 12 weeks later when I miscarried. I lay on the table at the hospital waiting to have a DNC and wondered how this could happen. I already have three healthy children and this has never happened before, my heart was breaking.

Brad and I decided we should wait a few more months before trying again, but God had other plans.

Two months later we discovered I was pregnant again. I was in shock and terrified. I spent week after week wondering and waiting. I was overjoyed when I made it to 8, 12, and then 16 weeks. I finally felt as though my dreams were coming true, I was really going to have another baby.

I began to get so excited, planning and dreaming about our future with four children, could I really do this, was I capable?

I never had the chance to find out if I was capable because my sweet little girl, Bethany Hope, was stillborn. I was left feeling lost and confused. We had spent so much time in prayer praying for God's will, praying for God to lead us in the right direction.

Now what?

I thought God had answered our prayers and now I'm left with no baby, nothing has changed and yet everything has changed.

For a while I could not understand why I felt so strongly that we were meant to have another child only to miscarry one baby and bury the other. The only answer my heart can grasp is that God has a plan.

I was meant to have my fourth child, whatever the reason may be. God does not make mistakes and He answers our prayers; yes, Bethany was a gift and an answered prayer. Children are a gift from God and God gave me Bethany Hope for a reason, I have to trust in that and cling to Gods ultimate grace to get through!

Father, thank you for loving me unconditionally! Thank you for answering my prayers even when they don't turn out the way I thought they would. Lord your plans are far greater than mine. Amen.

~Many times the plans or directions we feel that God is leading us to, do not turn out the way we imagine, but does that mean they are not part of God's plan? I know that God does not make mistakes and ALL life comes from Christ. Your child has a plan and a purpose and your child was meant to be – never forget that. When our life takes a wrong turn in our eyes, it might just be a right turn in the direction of Gods.

Day 6-Emptiness

"My grace is sufficient for you, for My power is made perfect in your weakness". 2 Corinthians 12:9

Today my sweet little Bethany Hope would have been 2 weeks old. I find myself wandering around aimlessly playing out what life would be like if she were still here. I wonder how I might juggle the responsibility of four children or how exhausted I would be.

I start cleaning the kitchen, trying to find something, anything to distract my ever wandering thoughts and I begin sobbing with tears of anger. I should be rushing to get house work done because Bethany will wake up any minute and need a new diaper or need to eat; but wait; I'm quickly reminded by my breaking heart that there is no baby to care for.

I long to hold her, nurse her, love her; honestly, I just long to have her back! I feel empty in a way I never dreamed would be a reality.

I'm lost and alone, or at least I feel alone.

Where is my Savior who is supposed to guide me and protect me from this kind of pain? My mind is racing with questions and my heart feels so empty. I fall asleep at night wishing she were here and I wake up praying this was all a bad nightmare!

I wonder if I wanted her too much...was I being greedy or selfish for wanting more children? I am running on a never ending treadmill of emotions right now and I am getting nowhere.

I walk around wondering how my life can seem so full and yet my heart can feel so empty. I desperately want to open my arms to those around me reaching out to love me and help me, but I just can't. I find myself just sitting and staring into space feeling more and more lost every day.

I can feel my Lord and Savior holding me in His arms and leading me day by day. I might not understand what is going on in my life right now, but I will lean into His arms and cry myself to sleep knowing that He will guide me through day by day!

My mother once told me that if we never sailed into the storms of life then why would we ever need a Savior? She's right! I do need a Savior because the storms of life are inevitable and I can't get through them alone. My Lord is my anchor and I choose to hold on tight and remind myself that He knows my deepest fears and thoughts. He knows how deeply my heart is broken. He knows how empty I feel and He is there ready to remove this emptiness from my heart.

Allow God to wrap you in His arms, He will guide you, comfort you, and collect every tear you shed. YES, He loves you and me that much! Cling to a Savior who can give you the rest your heart and soul need and allow Him to take complete control of your heart right now.

Father, emptiness fills my soul and you sweep in and fill my entire being day after day. Thank you for loving me!

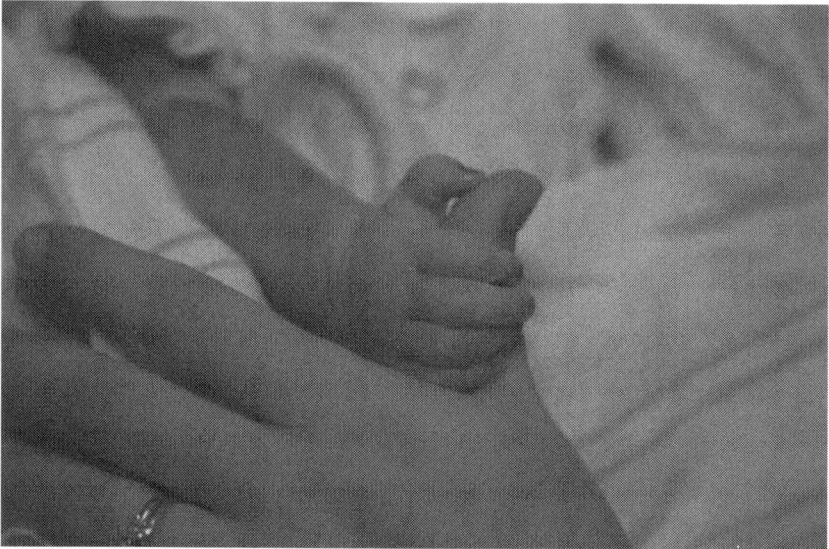

~Be patient in the grieving process and remember to be patient as you begin to work through your feelings of anger, depression, guilt, and sorrow. Never feel ashamed for what you feel and never think twice if you feel like you need to seek additional help from a therapist or support groups. Expressing your feelings of sorrow does not lessen your pain, but it does allow you to work through your feelings and allow your heart to heal. Write down how you are hurting today?

_____

_____

_____

_____

_____

_____

_____

_____

_____

_____

_____

_____

_____

_____

_____

_____

_____

_____

_____

_____

_____

_____

_____

_____

_____

_____

_____

_____

_____

_____

_____

Day 7-Broken plans

"Trust in the Lord with all your heart and lean not to your own understanding; in all your ways acknowledge Him and He will direct your paths."

Proverbs 3:5-6

I lie helpless in my Father's arms, awaiting and praying for Him to lead me in the right direction. I am surrounded by love and still feel so empty. I look aimlessly out the window as my neighbor mows his grass and cars drive by and think to myself, "How dare they".

It angers me to think that the world around me simply continues to go on through the day to day rotations of life while I sit here and wonder why life as I had planned it has been shattered and crushed. My heart is going a mile a minute searching for some kind of answer, some kind of reason as to why I had to be the one to lose a child.

I don't want to be that strong God!

I look to where Bethany Hope's cradle was so carefully set up only a few short weeks ago, and now stands a blank opening against the wall with no cradle and no baby.

I anxiously hope the phone will ring with Bethany's autopsy report thinking that this will settle my mind.

It amazes me how God can daily bring me to my knees searching, pleading, and begging for some array of light at the end of this dark tunnel.

"Life as I had planned it", well there's a little bit of humility thrown into the mix.

"I" am not in control. "I" am not in charge of my life or my children's.

I am learning that in the midst of tragedy we all look for short, fast answers because we think that will make the healing easier or maybe make the hurt go away a little faster. I am starting to realize that I might never get an answer as to why my little girl is now in heaven, however; there is one answer that always seems to come to mind in the middle of grief and that is to fix my eyes upon Jesus, hold on tight, and don't let go!

I have often heard people say that Jesus will never give you more then you can handle; I disagree. In fact, I know this is wrong because I guarantee you this is way more than I can handle on my own. If Jesus never gave us more then we could handle then why would we need Him? I know that I need Him to get through this daily battle in my life right now.

Although my body aches with pain, Jesus is pulling me through day by day showing me that He has a plan and a purpose for my life. My vision is blurred when I try and picture how any of this could possibly fit into God's purpose for me, but I know that without Him lifting me up each and every minute of the day right now, I would be broken and wounded, lying on the ground in sorrow.

Allow God to wrap you tightly in His arms right now. He freely comforts and loves you even when you are feeling completely unlovable!

Father, Allow me to trust in your guidance and your direction for my life. Allow me to completely trust you with all of my heart and lean not on my own understanding. Amen.

~Allow yourself to feel helpless and numb or whatever emotion you might be feeling. Your emotions will range from high to low or happy to sad, and all in the mix of one day. This is all normal and part of the grieving process. When you feel completely helpless, lie helpless in Jesus arms. Where are your feelings today?

Day 8-Rest

"Come to me, all you who are weary and burdened, and I will give you rest."

Matthew 11:28

I feel as though I am on a never-ending emotional rollercoaster and I can't find the bright red emergency stop! One minute I am up and the next minute I am sobbing like a baby.

I can still feel the physical pain of my milk drying up and it simply brings me to my knees. It is so hard to recover from a delivery when it constantly reminds me of my sweet daughter who is in heaven. My heart aches and I long to nurse her. I so desperately want to scream out how unfair this really is, but I just can't!

Life is not fair and God never promised it would be, but He did promise to protect us and heal our hearts. I daily have to remind myself of God's unfailing love and devotion to me. I also have to remind myself that I can scream at God and tell Him how unfair I feel this is; it's ok!

I sometimes pray for God to simply give me that extra little push to even make it through the day. I am longing for rest right now. I am longing for this feeling to go away and for life to be normal again. I am not even sure what normal feels like. I just can't even think anymore, it's as if I have no feelings left at all, I'm empty!

It is so easy to allow myself to take the path of "unfairness", knowing it will get me nowhere. I question myself daily on what signs I might have missed and I wonder if I could have done something different. In other words, I'm trying to play God! I can't go backwards. I can't blame myself.

I have to trust that God is holding me in His arms and is lifting me up day by day.

I often imagine Bethany running into my arms at the gate of Heaven smiling and saying, "Mommy, mommy, I'm so glad you're here!" Until then, I find comfort knowing that she is safe in the arms of my Heavenly Father, who will love her and take better care of her than I could ever imagine. She is happy, she is not in pain, and she and I will be united again. Praise the Lord! God's plate is never full and He wants you to hand your sorrows over to Him. He can and will deliver you from this moment in your life.

Father, I need that extra little push today. I need you're your arms to wrap so tightly around me that I feel your love in every direction I turn. My eyes are swollen from tears and my heart is aching, I need you Father. Amen.

~God never promises us a life free of pain, but He will guide us through our hurt and I believe He will use that hurt and pain in our lives to one day comfort others. You are not to blame for your child's death, and you can be rest assured that your sweet baby is safe and sound in the arms of Jesus Christ. How do you need reassurance today? How do you need rest today? "Praise be to the God and Father of our Lord Jesus Christ, the Father of compassion and the God of all comfort, who comforts us in all our troubles, so that we can comfort those in any trouble with the comfort we ourselves receive from God." 2 Corinthians 3-4

Day 9-Lost Memories

"Answer me speedily, O LORD; My spirit fails! Do not hide our face from me, Unless I be like those who go down into the pit. Cause me to hear Your loving kindness in the morning, For in You do I trust; Cause me to know the way in which I should walk, For I lift up my soul to You."

Psalm 143:7-8

I walked into the nursery today and quickly found myself on my knees before the Lord. I looked around at the diapers, blankets, changing table, lotions, car seat, and crib, and I wept with sorrow.

We had everything we needed to care for Bethany except for her.

My heart is crying out in pain and begging for something to change or be different. My spirit is slipping away day by day and my other children are longing to have their mother back.

I am taken back in my memory to the moment Bethany was born. There were nurses standing around, a baby bed ready for Bethany, my doctor encouraging me to push, my husband standing by being so strong for me and yet dying on the inside, and yet nothing was normal about this delivery.

Everyone in the room sobbed with tears of hopelessness, knowing that the precious little life that was coming into this world had already left this world to take her place in heaven. I am told that as soon as she was born my husband fell to his knees beside me sobbing as he held my hand.

I think of this moment that will forever be sketched in our hearts and I'm brought back to this moment weeks later sitting on the floor in an empty nursery wondering, what went wrong?

What did I miss?

Was there some sign that she was slipping away and I did not see it or feel it? I can quickly continue to go down the path of self pity and guilt while playing the "what if" game all day long, but knowing it will not get me anywhere and speaks no truth.

I did nothing wrong.

I could not have seen what was going to happen and my Lord and Savior will get me through this by reminding me day by day and minute by minute, that although I cannot change the dreadful past of what has happened, I can allow Him to lead me through and pick me up when I'm too weak to walk. God is never too weak to hold us. Allow God to give you strength and pick you up in His arms today.

Father, My Spirit fails me. Please give me the strength I need to make it from day to day and to not sulk in self pity but to honor you and allow you to lift me up when I feel too weak. Amen.

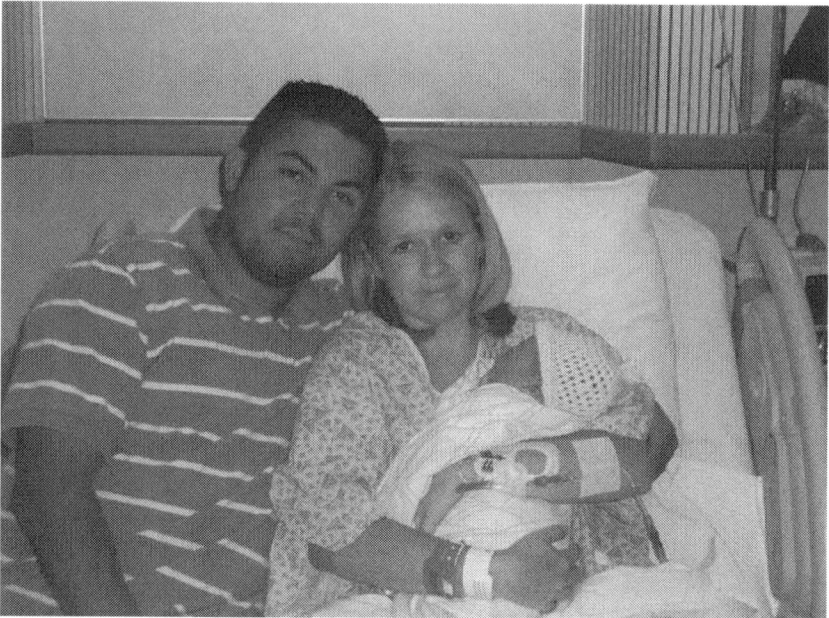

~I never wanted to forget the day or moment my daughter was born, these were the only memories I had of her besides my pregnancy. I compiled pictures and stories from throughout my pregnancy, the day she was born, and her funeral. I took these things and made a scrapbook for Bethany. Working on the book made me feel like I was doing something special in memory of my daughter. I love to look at the book when I miss her or want to show others my beautiful little girl. Where is your heart today?

_____
_____
_____
_____
_____
_____
_____
_____
_____
_____
_____
_____
_____
_____
_____
_____
_____
_____
_____
_____
_____
_____
_____
_____
_____
_____
_____
_____
_____
_____
_____
_____

Day 10-New Pain

"It is the Lord who goes before you. He will be with you; He will not fail you or forsake you. Do not fear or be dismayed."
Deuteronomy 31:8

I lay here in this hospital bed wondering if the last four weeks of my life are real. I am beginning to think I am watching myself in some crazy sci-fi movie and it is quickly spinning out of control.

About two days ago I began having some strange pains in my lower stomach. I assumed I was developing some sort of ovarian cyst or something; however; my mother could see the pain I was in and kept telling me I needed to see a doctor, but I refused.

It had only been three and half weeks since I lost Bethany and I really felt as if I were in survival mode. I was not going to the doctor. I was lucky to get out of bed. One night I was walking from my kitchen to the bedroom, which really is not that far, and by the time I made it to my bed I collapsed with tears streaming down my face.

My entire left leg was numb and my toes were tingling. I was scared. I went to bed praying for God to keep me safe and that I would go the doctor. The next morning I went to see my OB and she told me I needed to head to the ER for a full check up.

I was sitting in the waiting room wondering how stupid I was going to look when they told me nothing was wrong.

I had been in bed for three weeks taking every sleeping pill and anti-depressant my doctor would allow. I was really just trying to make it from day to day. After hours of waiting and one CAT scan later, my husband arrived just as I received the news.

The doctor looked at me and said,

"I have bad news. It's very serious and we're admitting you. You have a very large blood clot in your left leg".

By large he really meant a 15 inch blood clot going from my belly button all the way to my left knee, the technical term was DVT, or deep vein thrombosis.

The next morning I was being taken into surgery in what turned out to be a two week process of going in and out of my vein trying to remove this blood clot.

One early morning, about 2 in the morning, I burst into tears as the lab technician was drawing my blood from the bruises on my arm for the millionth time. She asked about a picture I had laying on the nightstand of my kids.

I realized how much I missed my family and how I was wasting my life sleeping away my grief. I realized that I wanted to live and I had about a million reasons too…or at least 4. I had a family at home who still needed a mom. I was determined to start living again and allow God to heal my heart.

I knew this was going to be a long journey, but I was ready to be anywhere other than a hospital at this point! My journey was truly only just beginning, although I could not see that at the time. I was surrounded by doctors and hospitals so much that everything was a daily reminder of Bethany; I just wanted to move on. Although the doctors could never completely get rid of my blood clot, I left the hospital with blood thinners and a new attitude. God was my healer and not the world. I was determined that God could cure my blood clot and my heart!

Father, you are the ultimate healer. Thank you for reminding me that you still have a purpose for me. Use me Lord to glorify you and your kingdom now and forever! Amen.

~Often times medical issues can and will arise after the loss of a child, especially a stillbirth. Spending time in and out of hospitals seeking answers can still often lead to disappointment and no answers. Allow Christ to carry your burdens for you when life seems too heavy. God has you in this journey and will be faithful to see you through? Are you struggling with a medical situation today? How and where do you need God's guidance in your life?

_____
_____
_____
_____
_____
_____
_____
_____
_____
_____
_____
_____
_____
_____
_____
_____
_____
_____
_____
_____
_____
_____
_____
_____
_____
_____
_____
_____
_____

Day 11–Learning to Dance in the Rain

"Consider it pure joy, my brothers, whenever you face trials of many kinds, because you know that the testing of your faith develops perseverance. Perseverance must finish its work so that you may be mature and complete, not lacking anything." James 1:2-8

I felt crippled as the paralyzing effects of the drugs began to set in; my body was tingling, my vision blurred and my heart numb.

I crawled into bed as my body melted into the covers and my pain and worries faded away into the darkness of the night.

I'm not sure exactly the mix of medicine I had taken, but I'm sure it consisted of my anti-depressant, sleep medicine, valium, 2 high doses of vicodin and one or two high doses of hydrocodone.

Killing myself was not my goal, but looking back it's amazing I survived the amount of pills I was taking. My goal was to numb the pain. It felt so good to not cry myself to sleep anymore, to not feel the hurt, to not question why God was making me go through something so extremely horrific.

Most nights I felt as though, without the medicine, my mind would race with questions and fears that would take over and I just couldn't take it anymore. I bottled my emotions and fears inside and forbade myself to talk to those who loved me the most; instead, I turned to prescription drugs to numb the pain.

After months of doing this and yelling at my husband when he accused me of being addicted, my Savior brought me to my knees.

I went to reach for the medicine one night and it was if Jesus Christ himself pulled it right from my hand and threw it on the counter. I fell in my hand crying and thought to myself, "What are you doing"?

I was sleeping everyday and missing out on life.

Taking pills and sleeping my days away are only temporary fixes, they simply numb the pain, not get rid of it.

I wanted more for my life. God allowed me to live through something that could have killed me: it is time for me to wake up and start living again!!! "I'm here for a reason"! God may have Bethany in heaven, but He is not quite ready for me. My time away from her is only temporary for I will see her again one day. I praise God for what I went through and for showing me that He is gracious and loving to the undeserving, and for that I am forever grateful! I know that life will not be easy and I will certainly still have bad days, but I am determined to allow Christ to work through me and use my life as a blessing to Him!

Father, thank you for ripping those pill bottles out of my hands. Thank you for showing me that in order to heal I had to let my heart work through the hurt and pain. Thank you for teaching me that life is not about waiting for the storms to pass, it's about learning to dance in the rain. Amen.

~Anti-depressants are perfectly normal and safe to take under a doctor's supervision. Do not feel ashamed if you feel like you need to take them in order to help you in your healing process. Abusing prescription drugs, however, can be very dangerous, so be careful and talk to your doctor about any and all medication you are taking. What are you fears today?

_____
_____
_____
_____
_____
_____
_____
_____
_____
_____
_____
_____
_____
_____
_____
_____
_____
_____
_____
_____
_____
_____
_____
_____
_____
_____
_____
_____
_____
_____
_____
_____
_____

Day 12-Strength

"So do not fear, for I am with you; do not be dismayed, for I am
your God. I will strengthen you and help you; I will uphold you
with my righteous right hand. "

Isaiah 41:10

How did I manage to get through yesterday, how do I get through today
or tomorrow; if I even get there! I am ready for God to heal my heart and
move past this moment in my life, but I am discovering that each and every
day is still a struggle and yet a gift.

I struggle with pain and questions and yet I also see what a precious
and miraculous gift life really is. Tomorrow is no guarantee for me or my
family, and yet what am I doing with today?

I feel as though I can do nothing, but with Christ I can do all
things.

Christ offers His strength but how do I accept something I'm not even
sure I want right now? Most days I wake up and feel as though I am some
alien in unfamiliar territory and I want to run as far as I can to find some
sense of normalcy, and on those days I realize that my strength does not
come to me, but through me. When I opened my heart and allowed God
to work it just amazed me what He was able to achieve. At some point
throughout this journey I have discovered that my only source of strength
and hope was through Jesus Christ.

This time in my life is ranked as a hopeless situation in which I was
ultimately a statue of silence, waiting on my Lord to take over! He feels
my pain today just as much as He felt my pain on the cross. God himself
watched as His only son was beaten and crucified for MY sins! I feel so

unworthy to be loved and lifted up by my savior, but what an amazing gift of grace He has shown me.

Are you willing to open your heart and accept this amazing gift of hope and grace? No amount of grief you or I can feel is any different than the grief God must have felt as He watched His only son be beaten and crucified to save the world. He knows our heart and feels our pain.

Father, grant me the strength to make it from day to day. You are the reason I can make it through today and made it past yesterday. Father you hold my future and I give my life to you. Hold me tight and lead me in your direction. Amen.

~Most days you might feel as though you have no strength at all to even accomplish the simple task that life requires. Christ can give you strength when you have nothing left. Open your heart today.

Day 13-Challenge

"Now to Him who is able to do immeasurably more than all we ask or imagine, according to His power that is at work within us." Ephesians 3:20

Challenge seems to be lurking around every corner I step these days. The physical challenge of making myself get out of bed or even using the bathroom, as if these things are even a necessity!

My leg is still sore and my heart is still broken. I want to move on and glorify God, but how? I want and understand that life must go on and my children and husband need me to be more than just a piece of lost art in this family, but this is such an overwhelming challenge these days.

I love my children, but feel like I push myself to be around them lately wondering, "Why was I allowed to keep them and will I still have them tomorrow?" I find myself fearful of every step they make, leaping at the faintest tumble or fall.

After realizing that my blood clot could have killed me, I wonder, "What's next or who's next?" I find myself watching and waiting for the next challenge to happen and it was not long before that challenge was once again staring me in the face.

I was holding my three year old son as blood was spraying from His head. He had tumbled down two bleachers at a baseball game (In an attempt to fly like superman), and landed on the ground.

I held His blood drenched face sobbing and thinking, God please don't take another child from me, please! Two stitches later I was beginning to see that Satan was attacking my heart. I was allowing him to make me feel frightened of life and what may or may not go wrong.

Life "IS" a challenge and challenge will be part of my life until eternity, I'm sure of it, but I cannot let it get the best of me. While it's no secret that the death of my child is the hardest challenge I have ever faced, it is also no secret that my Lord and Savior is stronger than any challenge that may come my way and He can use this challenge to ultimately strengthen me for His will, what an honor! My children will get hurt and there will continue to be suffering and challenges in this world, but there is hope and grace in Jesus Christ.

SO, if there are not already enough challenges in your life today, I challenge you to one more; get out of bed today and praise the Lord. Praise Him through this storm and allow Him to show you His amazing and unending grace! He IS able to more than we could ever ask or imagine, so step aside and allow Him to work through you today.

Father, grant me the wisdom and the strength to whole heartedly hand my fears and challenges over to you. Allow me to truly let go and let God! Amen.

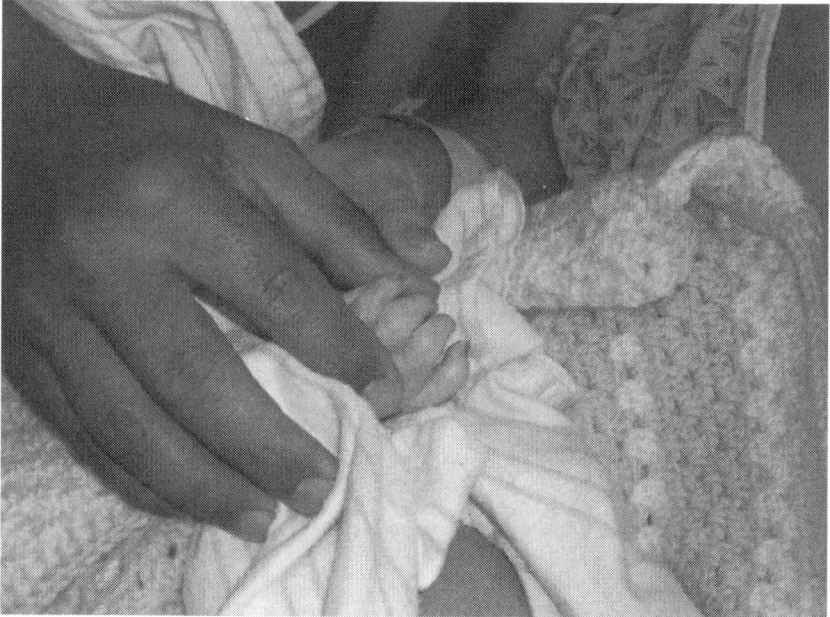

~Challenge will inevitably come your way, but you cannot live your life waiting for it to knock on your front door. List the things that challenge you the most and give yourself a goal to work through these challenges in your life. A big challenge for me was going into the nursery for the first time: it terrified me. Ask God to give you the strength you need to overcome your specific challenge.

Day 14-Lost

"Cast all your anxiety on Him because He cares for you."

1 Peter 5:7

I woke up this morning to the sounds of sweet little voices playing in the living room. I just laid in bed watching as my sweet three year old was cuddled up next to me slowly beginning to open his eyes. He looked up at me with a big smile on his face, kissed me gently, and then ran off to see what fun his Mimi and brother and sister must be having in the other room.

I found myself envious of his carefree spirit and overwhelming joy to start his day. With no urge or joy for myself to get out of bed, I simply laid there and listened. There was something inside me that wanted to smile and run out to enjoy the day with my children as if I was ready to have a good day; but my heart was not listening and decided to stay in bed.

Tears began to roll down my cheeks as I placed my hand across my stomach and looked down. Was it all a bad dream?

My belly is gone, but my arms are empty.

Where did the last nine months and my baby girl go? Was I even pregnant? Had I not felt her move and grow inside of me? Where do I go from here? One day she was here and the next day my world was undeniably changed forever! Her little face is forever embedded in my mind, my heart, and my life!

I cannot look for closure because I will never find closure. I will find happiness again through my Lord and Savior! However, I do not need to find closure because I will see my little girl again; playing in the streets of Heaven as if she were the prettiest angel in the world! if she where the prettiest angel in the world!

I cling to the fact that my life here is temporary and my life in Heaven is eternal. I will miss Bethany for a brief period of my life, but will have eternity to sing, play, laugh, and dance with her on the streets of Heaven. What an amazing gift to look forward to one day.

Father, help me to get through these days where I feel as though I can't even get out of bed. Oh how I miss my sweet girl. Give me the strength to make it from day to day when my mind is saying I can't go on. Thank you for your unending love. Amen.

~ Many days will come where you will lack the desire to even get out of bed, eat, or get dressed. Sometimes it feels as if it never even happened, and yet it did. Where is your heart today? Are you turning towards God during grief or blaming God for the sorrows in your life?

Day 15-Fear

"And we know that in all things God works for the good of those who love Him, who have been called according to His purpose."

Romans 8:28

There comes a time in life when we all become afraid or scared and fear can become overwhelming as it seeps into our souls and begins to take over.

I knew that Satan was attacking my heart, but I thought I had let go of this overwhelming fear until I learned that I was once again starting to become fearful of everything.

I was afraid to let my children get on the bus or even leave my side. I was frightened if my husband was late and forgot to call. I was spinning out of control and my poor family had to sit and watch.

My husband never knew what emotion he might get from me when he walked in the door. He must have been living on egg shells! I knew that I could not live like this, but the fear of losing one more person that I loved destroyed my inner being.

How do I move on?

How do I let go of this fear that has become so entangled in my life? I began to realize I have to make a choice, me or God?

I have to learn to let go, and Let God!

My pastor once asked me shortly after Bethany's death if I could say that I really trusted God. My first instinct was, of course I do, but then once I really thought about it I realized that although I do ultimately trust in God, I am not allowing Him to be in control of my life. I have no say in what tomorrow may bring, or whether or not I even make it to tomorrow,

HE is in control! The memories I have of my pregnancy and my daughter are forever etched in my mind. Dwelling in fear and sorrow will not take away those memories, but it will lead me down the road of unwanted fear and despair.

I am learning to allow God to use those memories for His glory and to place fear on the back burner. God loves me, and He is in control. I am ready to truly commit to believing that I really do trust Him. Are you ready to really let go of fear and open your heart to a God that wants only the best for you and freely gives us abundant grace whenever we ask?

Father, Please take this fear from my heart. Allow me to let go! Amen.

~ What are your fears? Why are you hurting today? Express your hurt and fears to a Savior who is ready to listen and lead you straight into His arms. Make a list of the fears holding you back in your life right now. Allow God to come into your life and take your fear away.

Day 16- Genuine Hurt

"I pray that out of His glorious riches He may strengthen you with power through His Spirit in your inner being, so that Christ may dwell in your hearts through faith."

Ephesians 3:16-17

Sometimes I imagine that the last few months did not happen, and other days I feel like I am regressing in pain and my heart is breaking even more. Although I continue to falter and fail through life as I selfishly battle my own desires over God's, my Lord never lets go of my hand.

He holds me so tightly while secretly whispering in my ear that He loves me and I will get through this. There are still days when I simply lack the strength or will power to even wash my own hair.

I can remember sitting on the side of the bathtub staring into the mirror and wondering whose reflection I was seeing. I was so lost and empty, or least that's what my reflection was revealing to me. "I want more," I thought! I don't want to be this lost soul deteriorating right before my family. I want to let Christ take over and honestly, I had no other choice.

I have often said, "When you're laying flat on your back, you only have one place to look!"

My Lord, Jesus Christ was there all along just waiting for me to say, "Your will, not mine." He was waiting to take my reflection and turn it into a beautiful piece of art for His glory.

It's funny how the more I tried to heal or turn off my emotions, the more I realized that God was right there waiting to do it for me. I just have to let go and give Him complete control. I longed to be the wife and mother my family needed, I just didn't know how to be that person anymore. It was as if I was giving them a broken doll and asking them to continue to play with it like nothing was wrong.

I was forever stained with the blood of my daughter on my heart, I was broken! This had changed a part of my inner soul and I didn't know how to find "me" again.

Day by day, life would continue to move on without her here; it really was as if it had never happened, but it did. God allowed it to happen and now He is allowing me to turn to Him in ways I never imagined I would need to.

God has a way of getting our attention and making us see that no matter what storm may come our way, we must decide what umbrella we are going to hide under: our own or the umbrella of His wings?

My favorite thing to remember about being a Christian is that everyone falls, but it's how we choose to get back up that truly matters. Life will have obstacles and as Christians we will suffer, but we must decide to have faith in the Savior that is ultimately stronger than any tribulation. He simply wants us to rely on Him. Can you freely do that today? Whose umbrella are you carrying through the storm?

Father, I have fallen, been broken and crushed into a million pieces and yet, you picked me right back up and ever so gently put me back together again, amazing! I choose to stand under your wings and allow you to carry me through the storms of my life as often as they may come. Amen.

~There will periods during your grieving in which you feel like you are doing better and then periods in which you feel like you are starting all over. Although these times may come and go, remember there is no time table when healing over the loss of a child. Your heart is broken and only God can rebuild your life if you allow Him. Remember to stay under the wings of Jesus Christ and give your heart time to heal. What are you feeling today?

_____

_____

_____

_____

_____

_____

_____

_____

_____

_____

_____

_____

_____

_____

_____

_____

_____

_____

_____

_____

_____

_____

_____

_____

_____

_____

_____

_____

_____

_____

Day 17-My Heavy Heart

"The Lord is a refuge for the oppressed, a stronghold in times of trouble."

Psalm 9:9-10

My body somehow managed to get out of bed this morning, although my mind was far from ready to get up. I felt like a robot as I marched around the house getting everyone ready for the day.

Amazingly, the big kids made it to school and my little man made it to preschool, my duties were done and I had only been awake for two hours, now what?

My heart felt so empty this particular day that I could hardly even bring myself to think one single thought.

As I looked around the quiet house all I could focus on were the breakfast dishes still on the table, toys all over the floor, and a sky high pile of laundry waiting on me to take charge. I thought, "If I just close my eyes it will all go Away?"

Sadly, closing my eyes changed nothing around me. I decided to lie down on the couch and quickly dosed off in to what turned in to a three hour nap.

I woke up sweating and somewhat confused about where I was. I must have been dreaming because I jumped up thinking my baby was crying and I had overslept.

I suddenly found myself standing in the center of the room looking around at the same mess I had fallen asleep to and the chilling silence which surrounded me.

I felt weak in my knees.

My heart began to pound and I could feel the tears swelling in my eyes as it become harder and harder to breathe! Anger began to fill my entire soul as I cried out,

"Why"!

The anger that was filling my body was taking over, and I did not like this feeling at all! I then cried out for God to take over and take this anger away. I verbally prayed out loud to my Heavenly Father, expressing my anger and I allowed Him to lift these feelings away.

I decided right then and there that GOD is in control and allowing Him to harvest all of my fears and feelings had to be better than this overwhelming anger taking over. I freely expressed my anger and gave it to God and I chose to live for Him and trust that He has the best intentions for my life. I will allow Him to show me hope for a new day.

It's amazing how God works when we let Him. I got up from the floor and to my surprise I was ready to take on the day and the so called "mess" around me. I realized that it is because of God I can clean up after the ones I love and sacrifice my time to take care of them and provide them with a clean home. It's ok to be angry, even at my Savior, but are you harvesting that anger or giving it to God?

Father, thank you for hearing my prayers. Thank you for letting me scream and be angry. Thank you for carrying my burdens so I don't have to. Thank you. Amen

~Anger is a normal part of the grieving process, but many times can be hard to understand. I had a hard time accepting that I could be angry with God and yet still love Him. Keeping anger inside can be unhealthy and often times keep you from healing. Let your anger out and give it to God. How are you angry today? God wants you to communicate your anger with Him.

Day 18-Empty Guilt

"Finally, brethren, whatsoever things are true, whatsoever things are honest, whatsoever things are just, whatsoever things are pure, whatsoever things are lovely, whatsoever things are of good report; if there be any virtue, and if there be any praise, think on these things." Philippians 4:8

I struggle sometimes in drowning out my own selfish desires and thoughts with what God is trying to reveal to me. It is much easier to simply fade away into the darkness and consume myself with sorrow and guilt.

Guilt and blame are some of the strongest emotions I have had since Bethany's death. Guilt of wanting her too badly, putting my desire for her above God, and blaming myself for her death.

I remember having a few contractions and some "strange" pains, the night before I realized she was gone. I remember her moving quite a bit that night and I was very uncomfortable and tired. I had taken some doctor prescribed pain medicine and went to sleep.

I only wish I had known then that that would be the last time that I would feel her move.

I struggled for months, thinking and wishing I had gone to the doctor that night.

My mind has been like a broken puzzle and I just can't seem to put the pieces together.

I felt overwhelming guilt for taking my pregnancy for granted and not being grateful for every day, every kick, and every moment I was blessed to have her inside of me.

The more I replayed those last few days over and over again the guilt was beginning to overwhelm me when I finally realized that it was false guilt! Guilt is a feeling of being responsible for an offense or crime. I had not committed any offense or crime.

My doctor had assured me many times that even if I had gone to the doctor they probably would have sent me home. There was no way of knowing her heart would just simply stop beating.

Ultimately blaming myself and consuming myself in guilt takes away from the joy Jesus Christ has in store. He knew this would happen; He knew I would get through this, and He knew it was not my fault but His will for me to trust in Him!

Stop feeling guilty and allow God to truly show you a peace like no other. Believe that He had and has a plan for you and guilt is not part of that plan. You are not to blame and you did not cause this pain in your life, but GOD can and will use this time to bring you closer and closer into His arms; how magnificent.

Father, thank you for wrapping your arms so tightly around me tonight. Please take away this guilt that is eating away at my heart. I know deep down I did nothing wrong and this guilt I am feeling is false guilt, so please rid me of this pain and sorrow. Amen.

~Guilt is such an easy emotion for a mother to take on after the loss of her child. As mothers, we question our every move, every breath, and every mistake as a possibility that we could have done something different to save our child. These are not feelings of guilt, but more so our way of searching for some kind of answer to the unknown. Remember, this is empty guilt and not real guilt. Write down the things you are feeling guilty about and pray for God to help you see these things as false guilt and not real.

_____

_____

_____

_____

_____

Day 19-Regret or Joy

"Light is shed upon the righteous and joy on the upright in heart." Psalm 97:11

I find myself missing my little girl so deeply today and wondering why life can be scary, lonely and completely unpredictable! Saying goodbye to my child is not the way it was supposed to be. No parent should have to plan their own child's funeral. I have done what feels like the impossible....my heart is breaking.

I am struggling with why things seem so backwards in my own life? My daughter should be reflecting on my life one day, not me sitting here wondering about all of the wonderful things she could have been. I am 29 years old and I am going through what no mother should ever have to feel, I'm letting go and saying good bye to a life I never even got to know outside of my womb and yet a life I was head over heels in love with!

I am taken back to the exciting moments of finding out I was pregnant. The moment where nothing else seems to matter and my heart might jump out of my chest with excitement. I can still remember the butterflies in my stomach as we went in for our first ultrasound. Seeing that cute little peanut with a strong flickering heart was a dream come true.

I can remember the first moments I felt her move and then the nights she moved so much I could not sleep. I loved the excitement of my children's little faces when they could feel her little body moving inside mommy's ever growing tummy.

These exciting and fond memories of my pregnancy are starting to seem somewhat trivial now, or are they?

I have wonderful and vivid memories of my time with my daughter, right down to taking a nap with her the day she was born. Was I supposed to forget the moments I had with her, pack them away in a box as if she never existed?

I asked myself, if I could go back to the early moments of my pregnancy and God gave me the choice of losing her then or carrying her full term and losing her the way I did, what would I choose?

I realized that I would do it all again just for those precious memories I have with her. I would not change those moments or the lessons God is teaching me through this for anything!

I am not going to pack her or my memories away. She is part of my life, my heart, and my story for as long as I live, and I will never let go of the joy God is bringing into my life through the life of my little angel, Bethany Hope!

Father, Thank you for the memories I have with my daughter. They are memories I will cherish and love forever. Thank you for reminding me that life is precious and to never take any moment we are given for granted. Amen.

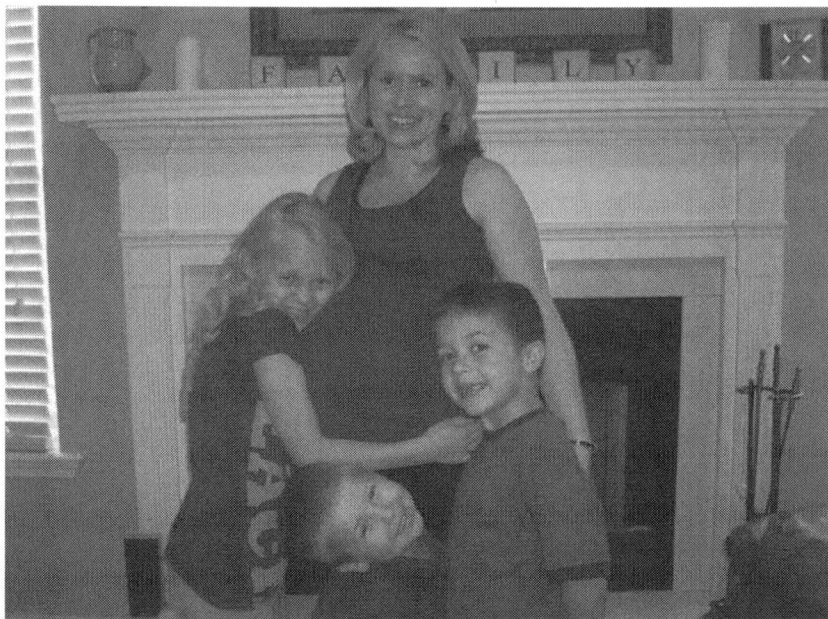

~Many times your family, friends and the world around you can make you feel as though you are supposed to just heal and pack away your baby and their memories in a box. The time your baby spent growing inside of you are precious memories that only you can hold. Write down the good times you remember with your baby and from your pregnancy. Hold on to those memories as precious times.

_____

_____

_____

_____

_____

_____

_____

_____

_____

_____

_____

_____

_____

_____

_____

_____

_____

_____

_____

_____

_____

_____

_____

_____

_____

_____

_____

_____

_____

_____

_____

_____

_____

_____

_____

_____

_____

_____

Day 20-Faith

"If you have faith as small as a mustard seed, you can say to this mulberry tree, 'Be uprooted and planted in the sea,' and it will obey you." Luke 17:6

Faith? Is this just a word in your vocabulary or do you really know what it means to have faith?

This so called Faith is something my heart has really began to ponder over the last few months. For years I was someone who proclaimed to have great faith and encouraged others to just have faith. I can remember talking to friends who might have been having a bad day and I would tell them that if you really trust in Christ then just have faith for Him to work things out.

WOAH, did I ever get a wakeup call on my so called faith. It was not until my little girl went to Heaven and my world came crashing down around me that my "faith" was finally put to the test.

Now, don't get me wrong, I was no stranger to heart ache! There had been many times in my life where I felt completely lost and I knew that Christ was the only way to get me through, have faith, right?

Well, I have to say, no heart ache I had ever been through before compared to planning a funeral for a child that I had carried for nine months, sacrificing my body to give this child the perfect place to grow into this perfect little miracle. This kind of heart ache demanded a whole new kind of faith, or did it?

Faith is faith, right?

The months following my daughter's death were anything but easy. I had days and even moments where I would beg God to just push me throughout the day. I have had moments of fear, anger, guilt, and even regret, but now looking back at those moments I can see that I did turn to Christ and He DID pull me through, every single time I needed Him to!

I am strongly standing on two feet and allowing God to lead my life in His direction, and I will praise Him no matter what may come my way. I finally got an answer to my question; faith is hoping for things that cannot be seen but are very true and real in the presence of God.

Faith is easy to have when things seem great around us. It's when we fall to our knees that we make the decision: Do we really believe what we say we believe?

My answer in easy, yes! I do have faith for my Savior to comfort me and protect me no matter what life brings my way and my proof lies in the fact that I am learning and growing in Christ more at this time in my life than ever before! Where does your faith lie?

Father, thank you for reminding me that my faith lies in you and you alone. Help me day by day as my faith is put to the test! Thank you Father for showing me how much I needed you! Amen.

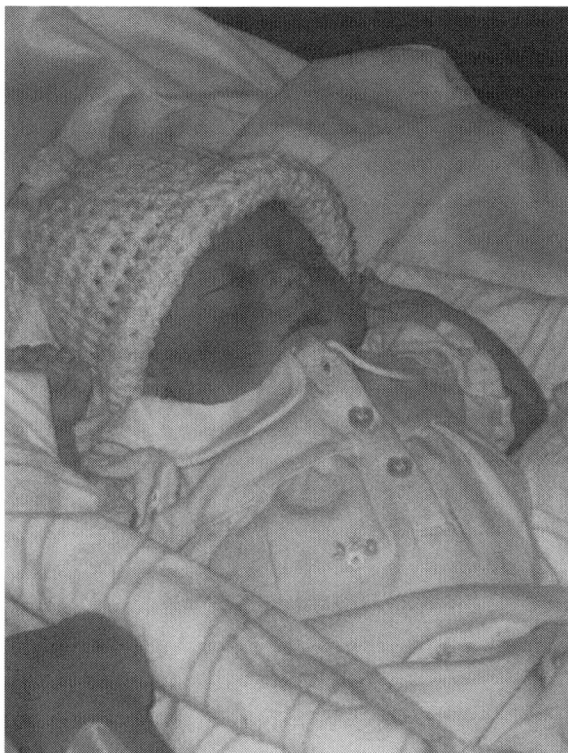

~Faith can be a hard concept to really understand and it can be difficult to commit to allowing Jesus Christ to pick up the pieces of our broken lives. Where is your faith today? Are you willing to have faith that Jesus Christ can pull you through the darkest of days and has great plans for your future? Where do you stand today?

Day 21-Bitterness

"Suffering causes bitterness to people who do not understand problem solving devices, principles, and give number one priority to their relationship with God."

Deut. 32:24

I have not been sleeping very well these last few days, weeks, even months. I find myself feeling so very lost and wondering what it is God wants from me. I read my Bible over and over again saying and doing all of the so called "right" things.

I find myself starting to doubt Gods word and frankly, this terrifies me! I am trusting that my life is in His hands and that His plans are far more glorious than my own, but why am I still aching and burning with grief inside?

Why are there days that I CAN'T stand to see someone walk by holding a baby girl without completely falling apart? Why do I get so angry when people ask me if we are having more children and I want to scream at them to GO AWAY? Bitterness! Bitterness is a devastating feeling which can quickly spiral out of control into feelings of hatred, cruelty, and self-pity. A bitter person will become withdrawn and afraid of everything around them.

I realized that I was this bitter person. I was angry with others happiness and joy. I was mad because I was still hurting inside. I do not want to be bitter and angry, but how do I differentiate these feelings of bitterness with feelings of true sadness. I am learning that this battle is a daily battle, but I am not alone. God is willing to fight this one for me if I can just let go!

I have to understand that my heart will always ache for my daughter, but Gods grace and love will continually fill up my life.

I might fall apart weekly if not daily, but I also know that my Savior is there to pick me back up again, day after day, after day! Suffering can turn into bitterness without turning your suffering over to Christ and allowing Him to work through your hurt and pain.

I now know what God wants from me: faith and a trusting heart that He is guiding me and loving me through every minute of my life. He is waiting with open arms to embrace my fears and daily challenges, which will inevitably come! I AM NOT ALONE!

Father, forgive me for the bitterness in my heart. Allow me to turn away from being bitter and turn to you. Amen.

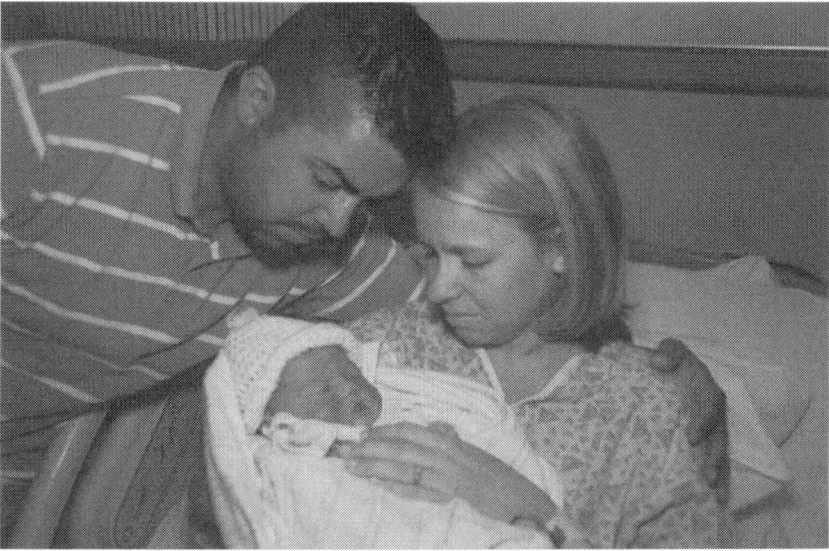

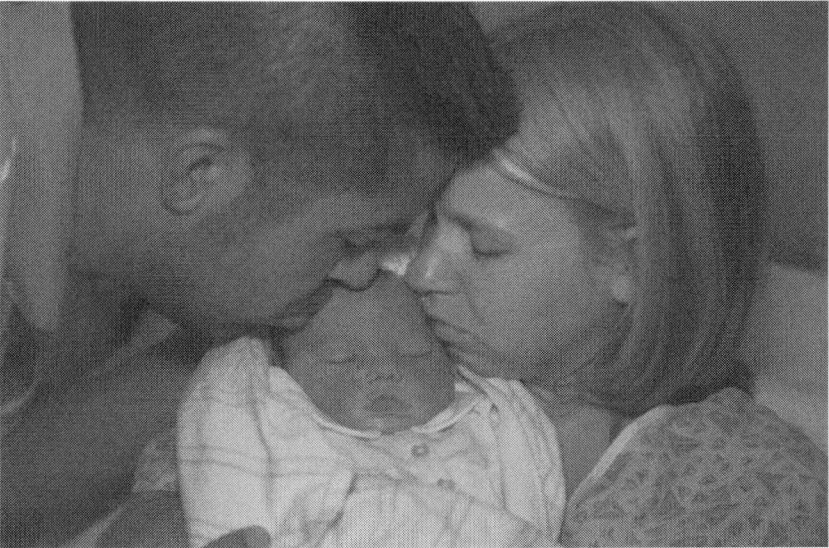

~ When trouble comes your way you can choose to be bitter or get better through Christ, which do you choose today? Where is your heart today? What bitterness are you holding onto?

Day 22-Blessings

"You, O Lord, keep my lamp burning; my God turns my darkness into light." Psalm 18:28

My insides are screaming to be set free. Part of me wants to run as far as I can into the deepest darkest hole where no one can find me! I feel as though my life is spinning out of control and no matter how fast I run, I just can't catch up.

How can I feel on top of the world one day and the next, completely broken and useless? I take one step forward and two steps back.

Will I ever be normal or whole again?

There is a hole in my heart and I am not sure I will ever be the same. I feel so separated from my children, my husband, and at times my Savior. I cry out for my Lord to scoop me up in His arms and make all of the pain go away.

For years, I would half-heartedly sympathize with women who went through a miscarriage or the loss of a child. I would think, "How sad, I can't even imagine!" The truth is; I was right! I could not imagine at that time in my life how horrific this kind of loss really is. I had no clue that my heart could be completely broken and my entire being so instantly changed forever.

Will there ever come a day when I don't wonder, what if, or what might have been? I still imagine what my life would be like if Bethany were still here. I imagine my other children loving her and my husband falling asleep with her on the couch. I am suffering in ways that just do not seem fair, in fact, they seem cruel! Why has my heart been crushed into a million pieces?

Children are a gift from God and yet my gift has been taken, along with my heart. As I'm writing this, I am watching my children playing not so peacefully together on the floor, and I am reminded that God's blessing can come in many different packages. The truth is; I am blessed! I would not trade those priceless little arguing children for anything in this world.

God has allowed me to go through the most unimaginable trauma possible, but through it I am learning to see the blessings in my life. Although many days are a complete struggle, I also know that grief takes time and along with God's amazing grace and love I will overcome, you will overcome! I might continue to take steps backwards, but I also know that God will continue to push me forward and grant me the will to see the blessings in my life even through the darkness!

Father, forgive me for the anger I have towards others in my time of grief. Thank you for reminding me that I am blessed and even through the struggles I must rejoice in what I have. Thank you for loving me through my pain. Amen.

~ Is your broken heart blinding you to the blessings you have in your life? Are you angry at the blessings others around you seem to have? How can you turn your anger towards others into love?

_____
_____
_____
_____
_____
_____
_____
_____
_____
_____
_____
_____
_____
_____
_____
_____
_____
_____
_____
_____
_____
_____
_____
_____
_____
_____
_____
_____
_____
_____
_____
_____
_____
_____
_____
_____
_____
_____
_____
_____

Day 23~New Life

"The LORD is close to the brokenhearted and saves those who are crushed in spirit. A righteous man may have many troubles, but the LORD delivers Him from them all." Psalms 34:18-19

Why do so many women feel like they must conquer the world and be a real live super woman in the process? I'm finding myself feeling very overwhelmed with life this morning. My mind is going a mile a minute on the here and now that needs to be done; however my heart can't seem to let go of the many things I'm missing out on.

I imagined lying in bed dressing my sweet little girl after a bath. I long to hear her crying and rush to her side. I feel so robbed of my motherly duties and I'm broken that I can't get them back.

My heart is once again empty and so confused with life right now.

I felt as though God had given me another chance to see the joy at the end of a long dark tunnel as I recently discovered I was pregnant again. This is the second pregnancy I have had since my sweet girl went to Heaven only 9 months ago and this one is now ending as did the last.

I think there was a part of me that thought if I had another baby it would take away the pain, but I was wrong. Discovering I was pregnant brought up new feelings and fears I wasn't ready to face. I wondered why Bethany was gone but now there was new life.

I'm recalling the events of the last year of my life and wondering where to turn from here. I have had three miscarriages now and one stillbirth, maybe God is saying enough is enough. When has my heart been broken and torn to enough pieces? Part of me is looking, longing for life to be any kind of normal, really, just different than the last 9 months.

For so long I wanted an answer as to why I lost my little girl, and then

I just wanted to numb the pain. Many days I just wanted to pretend like nothing had gone wrong and life was normal. I found myself once again heading for the pill bottle and yet my hand froze on the cabinet door.

Taking extremely strong pain medicine that might allow me to sleep for tonight will only temporarily allow me to not hurt. I collapsed onto the kitchen counter as the tears began to flow from my eyes. I am running in all the wrong directions here. I am sleeping away the pain so I don't have to think about how bad it hurts when the truth is, God already knows! God already knows how deeply I'm hurting and is waiting for me to fall into His arms.

I have to deal with this pain; I have to accept that I can't go backwards. I can't bring my little girl back, but I can allow God to move me forward. I can allow Bethany to be part of my life. I can deal with this through my Lord and Savior Jesus Christ. No amount of pills or sleep can really take away the grief you are feeling.

Running is fine, but make sure you're running in the right direction. Turn to Christ and turn to those whom Christ has placed in your life to love you and help you – that is the only true drug that works!

Father, I fall into your arms again. My heart is breaking over losing yet another baby, and I just don't understand. I need you to give me strength and guidance. Heal my breaking heart. Lord, I 'm not sure how much more my heart can take. Father, hear my cries and save me from this darkness. Amen.

~Getting pregnant after the loss of a baby can be exciting for so many mothers and yet those who try to become pregnant without success can be facing a road to a deeper depression. Make sure you allow yourself to truly heal over your loss before committing to trying for another baby. Make sure you are ready and willing to travel down the road of the unknown. Allow Christ to lead your heart and guide you down this road. Remember you are never alone.

Day 24-Power

"Without Christ, I am powerless to do anything (John 15:5)."

I used to think that I was one of those people who could care less about being powerful or in charge of something. I would have labeled myself as simple, easy going, and carefree. In light of all I have been through, I am beginning to rethink my original assumptions of myself.

Ever since I was a little girl I would dream of being a wife and mother. I loved playing with my baby dolls and imaging being a real mommy one day. I wanted a big family and in my world life would be perfect, fairy tale perfect!

I think the most devastating part about my dreams was the fact that I really thought this kind of fairy tale was obtainable. I was not dreaming for wealth or riches, just a big happy family. Somewhere over the last few months I am wondering want went so wrong and where is this big happy family I wanted so badly? I do want to be in charge and I do want power, power to have as many happy healthy children as my heart can take, but does God want this for me? The problem with wanting to be in charge of our own lives is that often it leaves us so heartbroken when things do not go as WE planned.

I do have three children and I have a great life, so why oh why am I letting Satan make me feel as though I have nothing, when I have so much more then I really even deserve.

Wanting my own desires and becoming so self absorbed has left me with a very selfish heart. I struggle with why I wanted more when I know there are many women who would do anything to even have one child. Children are a blessing from God, so is it a crime to want more of a good thing?

My heart is aching and breaking for women who have gone through what I have and yet have no other children to find joy in, yet mine are right in front of me and I appear to be blind to what God has given me. UGH! What is wrong with me!!!

My heart is lost and my soul feels empty, but I am so blessed to know that I have a Savior that is ready and waiting to fill my soul with joy and contentment again. It just takes time: time to realize that without Christ I am powerless to move on and powerless to see the blessings through the pain.

I think my original assumptions of myself are correct. I am simple, easy going, and carefree, but I live in a world that is NOT, simple, easy going, or carefree, and I must learn to allow Christ to have the power in my life and give me the power to not conform to the world's idea of life.

Is wanting more of God's blessings a bad thing? No, as long as they are part of God's plan for your life. I am learning that, although I might have wanted a very large family, God is telling me to be content in the blessings I have. God has given me three children and if I don't wake up and start enjoying them now, I might be dealing with a whole new level of regret and I am not ready for that!

Father, forgive me for wanting so much control in my life. Thank you for making me see the blessings you have given me. Help me to hand my control over to you to lead my life. Amen.

~ What are the blessings in your life that are hiding behind the pain and sadness in your heart? Are you wanting control of your life or are you willing to hand the steering wheel over to your Lord and Savior? Who is in charge today?

_____
_____
_____
_____
_____
_____
_____
_____
_____
_____
_____
_____
_____
_____
_____
_____
_____
_____
_____
_____
_____
_____
_____
_____
_____
_____
_____
_____
_____
_____
_____
_____

Day 25– Confused

"Being confident of this, that He who began a good work in you will carry it on to completion until the day of Christ Jesus". Philippians 1:6

I feel as though I am back on that emotional rollercoaster and I am not sure where to go. My eyes are swollen from the tears that seem to uncontrollably stream from my eyes. These last days, weeks, well months really, are beginning to seem like a blur.

The harder I try to understand what God wants from me the harder I feel like I fail. I find myself lying face down on my floor today begging God to help me, give me some ray of light at the end of this dark tunnel.

After the last two miscarriages I had, both after Bethany, my husband decided to get another vasectomy. We spent a lot of time talking about this and both felt God saying it was best for us. I spent time praying about this on my own, and yes I felt God saying it was what we needed to do, but it still was so very hard.

It was hard to finalize never being pregnant again, never getting my happy ending, never nursing again, no more baby, ever! Deep down this really broke my heart, but I knew God was telling me this was right.

A week after Brad's surgery I was SHOCKED to find out I was pregnant again for the third time since we lost Bethany. I thought this was my gift from God, my sign. My doctor began HCG testing and by 5 weeks my levels were going down. Once again I was losing my baby.

Ok, roll call; 4 total miscarriages and 1 stillbirth.

I now have more children in Heaven than I do here. I am so lost. I went through with what I felt God was telling me to do, so why did I need to lose one more baby? Was it really necessary? I really feel as though my heart cannot take this rollercoaster ride anymore. I'm done!

I'm not sure why God allows things to happen the way He does, but I do know that He has been by my side the entire time. Maybe I just needed to know that I was done with the rollercoaster ride to confirm our decision to have the vasectomy done, or maybe I will never know.

I'm told by my pastor and counselor friends that everything I am feeling and questioning is very normal, but nothing about losing a child feels normal. Please tell me what feels normal about holding your dead child in your arms and burying them or cremating them; isn't it supposed to be the other way around? Who defines what normal is, anyways?

Life is not easy. God never promised it would be, but He did promise to never leave you. I have learned that my happy ending is not meant to be here on earth, but in heaven when I meet my Bethany Hope on the streets of heaven; that will be my happy ever after. One day my entire family will be together again. Until then, I praise God now and forever more.

Father, watch over my sweet angels above. Protect them and love them. I know life is not always easy, and my life seems so far from anyone's view of normal, but thank you for always staying by my side. Amen.

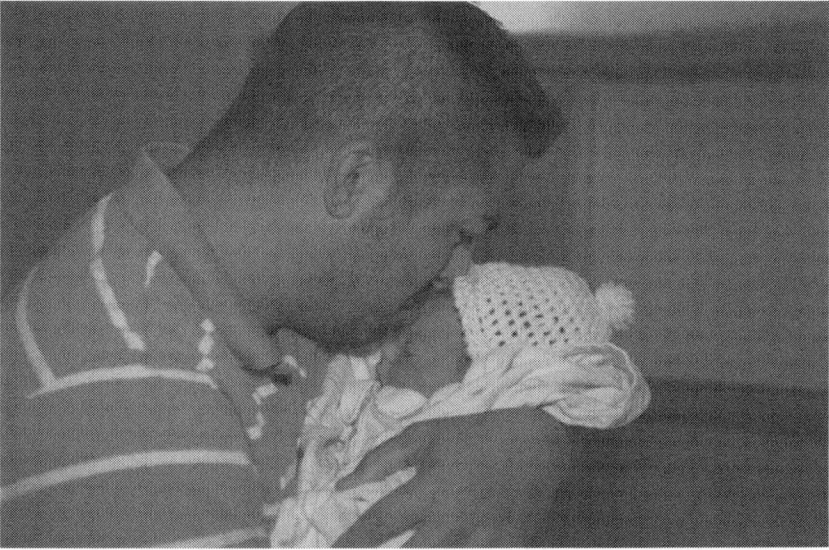

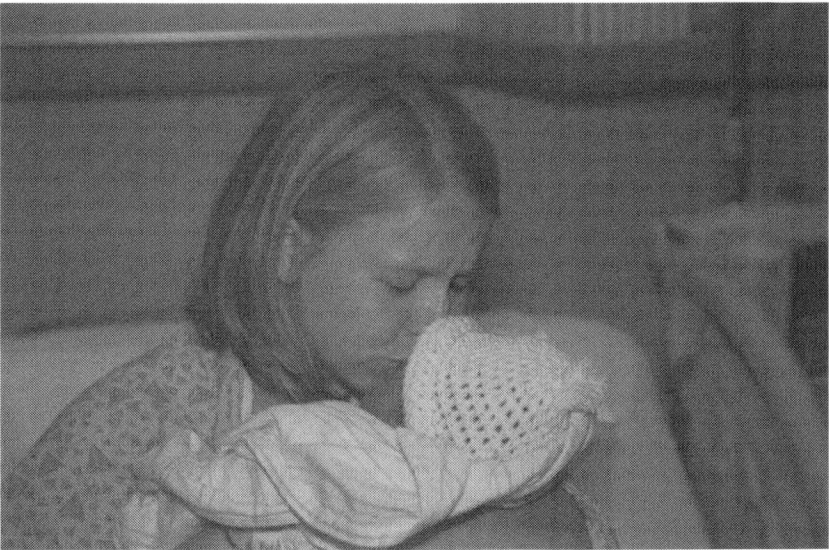

~Having multiple miscarriages can be challenging and overwhelming, especially after the death of another child. Please seek help and guidance and do not go through this alone. If you wish to add to your family and continue to suffer miscarriages, ask your doctor about genetic testing. Where is your heart today?

Day 26-Contentment

"I know what it is to be in need, and I know what it is to have plenty. I have learned the secret of being content in any and every situation . . . . I can do everything through Him who gives me strength." Philippians 4: 12-13

According to Webster's online dictionary, the word contentment means: happiness with one's situation in life.

I have really been thinking a lot about contentment these days and what it would mean for me to truly be content. I have recently discovered that someone I know has been struggling with infertility for years and has completely put her faith in Christ during such a difficult time in her life.

I have been walking around for weeks in survival mode just hoping I would wake up from this living nightmare I am so deeply embedded in and then I hear this story and I can't get it out of mind.

For years I have been focused on wanting more children and always wondering what tomorrow may bring, but what about today? I have wondered why I have had four miscarriages and why I lost my sweet little girl. My brain is completely drained of the thought we will actually have another child and then it hits me:

Be content!

Why do I waste my time worrying and planning out every detail of my life when my Lord and Savior has already done this for me? I have been blessed! I have a family that I am going to miss so much with because I am sulking in what I cannot have.

I think the hardest thing to hear as a Christian is when God answers us, but that answer is no. I don't know what tomorrow holds and I don't want to miss opportunities to love and spoil my family and yet that is what I am doing. God has given me an amazing life. He is showing me that

He will continue to turn the sorrow into joy and it is time I stop thinking about tomorrow or focusing on the past and be content in today. The plans my Savior has for me are better than any I could choose for myself...I am ready to be content in what God has given me!

Are you ready to place all fear and worry aside and be content in Jesus Christ today? Be content in what He has given you and praise Him no matter what the day may bring! One of my favorite songs is, *"Change My Heart Oh God."* I long to be more like my Heavenly Father because He modeled me in His image and has planned out every detail of my life according to His purpose. Are you ready to allow God to change your heart and let you shine as the amazing jewel He created you to be?

> Change my heart oh God Make it ever true
> Change my heart oh God May I be like You
> You are the potter I am the clay
> Mold me and make me This is what I pray!

Father, change my heart oh Lord and please make me more like you. Help me to be content in what you have given me today and not focus on what I do not have. Tomorrow may never come. Help me to live today by being content in all you have blessed me with. Amen.

~Contentment sounds so easy, but was so hard for me to come to grips with. It was hard for me to realize that God was actually saying I needed to be content with the family I had. As a mother I wanted more children and I wanted to be in control of that. I had to give that control to my Savior and learn to be content in the life He had given me, before I risk the loss of all joy in my life. What can you do to find contentment in your life today?

_____

_____

_____

_____

_____

_____

_____

_____

_____

_____

_____

_____

_____

_____

_____

_____

_____

_____

_____

_____

_____

_____

_____

_____

_____

_____

_____

_____

_____

_____

_____

_____

_____

_____

_____

Day 27-Jealousy

"By His light I walked through darkness." Job 29:3

I find myself wanting what others around me have, not material things, but motherly things. I long to be that mother of a newborn, or chasing myself in circles while pretending I'm good at balancing 3 kids, a newborn, a husband, and a house. I know I already have all of these things, except the newborn, but my heart just can't let go.

I am scared I am going to become so wrapped up in wanting my baby back that I am going to miss out on the precious gifts God has already given me. It's funny how life can slowly begin to change and we just wake up one day and realize we are this strange new person. I had not realized how much I have changed until the last few weeks.

My husband and I have been arguing like crazy and although neither of us is perfect, I can see that this arguing is stemming from so much change. I think that we have been going through the motions of everyday life pretending like nothing has changed when our entire world has been turned upside down.

I am struggling with the fact that he seems to be healing from all of this change must faster than me as if nothing has changed at all. I find myself angry and jealous of how easy it seems for him to just let go. I can feel myself pulling away from him and many others around me.

My mom will call and I know I sound like I am a million miles away. I can hear in her voice how she just wants to help me and make this pain all go away, and I just don't know how to let her help me. I know she feels so lost right now, and my husband, well I'm not even sure he knows who he's married to anymore.

I am beginning to ask myself if I am really allowing Christ to help me deal with this change in my life or if I am pushing those who love me away; while I fade into depression as if no one will ever understand where my heart is. At times I can't even talk about what I'm feeling, good or bad, because I can't seem to find the right words.

My husband is trying so hard to be there for me and to understand and I have just pushed him aside. God has reminded me tonight that change is part of life. I cannot consume myself with jealousy of what others have just because their lives appear free of change and challenge. I am blessed with a husband that still loves me, a mother who is dying to help me, a father and entire family who love me, friends and a church family; what more could I ask for? I am asking for God to help me conform to this change in my life and to accept the things I cannot change.

Father, allow me to follow you and put my trust in you. Help me to stop pulling away from those who love me and care for me. Show me that throughout all of the change in my life, you are constant and will never change or leave my side. Thank you for this very sweet reminder! Amen.

~Seeing other mothers with new babies can be one of the hardest challenges one can face after losing a baby. Your heart longs for what they have. God clearly states that jealousy is wrong and yet this was so hard for me to overcome because it just didn't seem fair. There comes a point where you have to decide to put jealousy away and be happy with what God has given you in your own life. Focus your time on what you have and not on what you do not. How can you work on changing your jealously today?

_____

_____

_____

_____

_____

_____

_____

_____

_____

_____

_____

_____

_____

_____

_____

_____

_____

_____

_____

_____

_____

_____

_____

_____

_____

_____

_____

_____

_____

_____

_____

Day 28- Hidden treasures

"Not only so, but we also rejoice in our sufferings, because
we know that suffering produces perseverance; perseverance,
character; and character, hope. And hope does not disappoint
us, because God has poured out His love into our hearts by the
Holy Spirit, whom He has given us." Romans 5:3-5

I was walking into the lab today in what seemed like a new normal part of
my life. I was once again having my arm stuck a million times just to find
the perfect vein so they could check my blood levels.

I was impatiently sitting in the cold sterile lab chair waiting as the
nurse was gathering her equipment. As I ran my fingers through my
quickly thinning hair, considering it was coming out in handfuls by this
point, I dropped my head and prayed that this would be the time. My
blood levels would finally be perfect and I could stop taking such a high
dose of blood thinners.

I must have had tears in my eyes because the nurse said, "Honey, are
you ok?" I said, "Yes, ma'am, I just really dislike being stuck with needles
week after week. I'm turning into some kind of ugly pin cushion!" When
on the inside what I really wanted to say was, "PLEASE LET THIS ALL
BE OVER!" I felt like everything from my sweet Bethany to this hospital
was a never ending nightmare. I felt like I was never going to move on
because it was following me day after day. I just wanted to at least try and
move on.

Well, somehow the sweet nurse starting talking with me and I shared
my story and, to my shock, she already knew! She said that she had a friend
in labor and delivery who had told her about my story. She went on to tell
me what an impact that day had had on all of the nurses and doctors.

She said they were all watching as our pastors came in to pray with us while I was in labor and how calm we all seemed even through the tears. She said the nurses would all sit at the outside desk and just cry as they watched people walk into our room. None of them could even talk to one another as they were grieving with us. She said they all watched in amazement as I cared for my daughter as if she was alive and breathing. The love they saw was simply amazing.

At first I wondered why our situation had made such a strong impact on those around us, I mean, I was not the first one to experience a stillbirth delivery at this hospital, and then it hit me. I never really realized how calm and peaceful it was that day in that hospital room. All I ever thought about were the tears flowing from my face.

Looking back, I now realize that what all of those nurses and doctors saw that day was the power of Christ. Through the hurt and tears, Christ was pouring His love and grace onto us that day and now look at all of those He has touched with His presence.

I thanked the lady that day for telling me what she knew and I left the hospital thanking God for using me in such a powerful way. God can and will use us in many ways and often times He uses others to get our attention. God can shine through our lives even when we feel as though we are falling apart. Allow God to shine through your broken heart and show others His unending love!

OH Father, thank you for shining so brightly on what seemed like such a dark day. Father, thank you for using our story to shine the brightness of your glory and grace on all those who surround us. What an honor to be part of YOUR story, thank you Father. Amen.

~It is still amazing to me how God has used our story. Open your heart to what God is trying to reveal to you about the loss of your child. Open your ears to what others may know. Where is your heart today?

_____

_____

_____

_____

_____

_____

_____

_____

_____

_____

_____

_____

_____

_____

_____

_____

_____

_____

_____

_____

_____

_____

_____

_____

_____

_____

_____

_____

_____

_____

_____

_____

_____

_____

_____

_____

_____

_____

_____

Day 29- Inspiration

"For I know the plans I have for you," says the Lord. "They are plans for good and not for disaster, to give you a future and a hope." Jeremiah 29:11

I had the joy of subbing in a 4 year old class today at my son's preschool. I say joy, but the truth is deep down, I did not want to go.

I had been painting my house all week and my body was beat! I was exhausted, but I said yes and went in with somewhat of a bad attitude. After spending the day with 10 little 4 year olds, my whole attitude had changed and I realized just why God had sent me into this specific classroom.

There was a sweet little boy in the class by the name of James. He has the biggest smile I have ever seen. He is kind to his friends, very helpful, and shares with everyone. He was quick to help me find things in the cabinet or tell me how his teacher ran the class.

He laughs as if the world is the best place to be. He has so much joy for life, which is such an inspiration because he has all of this joy through his wheelchair. He will never walk again and still awaits many surgeries to fix a problem with his spine. This sweet 4 year old has so many burdens to carry and yet all that shines from him is the love of Christ.

He spins with laughter in his chair at music time, enjoying the life that God has allowed him to have. What a true inspiration. I have watched his mother bringing him in and out of school for weeks. She smiles and laughs with him with nothing but love and hope shining through on her face. She is true inspiration to me that life is hard and we are not always dealt the hand of cards we might hope for, but God will bring us the greatest treasures in life when we trust in Him.

Instead of self-pity, start praying.

When you feel down pray for the person standing next to you; you don't know their story but God does. Turn pity into prayer and sadness into joy by opening your heart to Christ.

Being around James brought so much joy and laughter into my heart. He was such a blessing, showing me that throughout difficulty, God is using us to shine and reveal His ultimate Glory. Thank you, James, for being a light to shine on others. You have truly blessed my life!

Father, thank you for sending me exactly where I needed to be despite my willingness to go. Thank you for using the innocence of a child to remind me that life is worth living day by day with as much joy as we are given. Thank you! Amen.

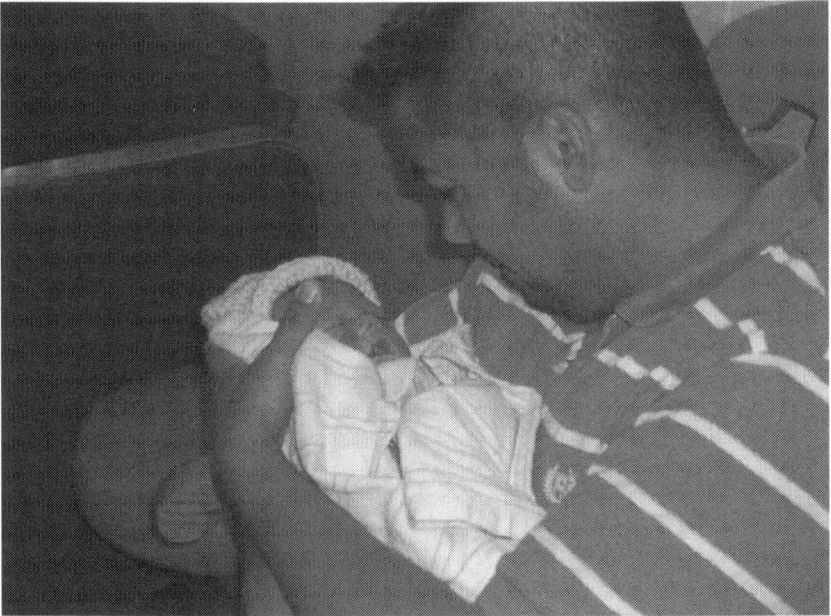

~Have you ever felt the nudge to go somewhere or do something and yet your heart was just not in it? Often times God is sending us exactly where we need to be and yet we resist because of our own insecurities. God can heal your heart in ways and through people you could never imagine. Open your heart to Christ and allow Him to work in your life today. Where is your heart today?

Day 30- Complete Restoration

"Restore unto me the joy of thy salvation; and uphold me with
thy free spirit"

Psalm 51:12

When we least expect it God can use our broken hearts in miraculous
ways. I had the honor of sitting in church this morning and watching my
husband give his testimony about our daughter, as pictures of her rolled
by on the screen above his head.

He spoke about a very special moment we had as we were both sitting
in the hospital bed holding our lifeless little girl the day she was born. She
had been with us all day and it was time to give her back to the nurse. Her
skin was cold and her lips were red. My body began to shake as I handed
her over to the nurse. I felt as though someone had just ripped out my
heart and was walking away, never to return. As the nurse left, I fell into
Brad's arms.

We were asking ourselves, "Where do we go from here, now what?"
Silence quickly filled the cold room as he gently started to sing the words
to a very familiar song:

"Restore to me The joy of your salvation. Restore to me The wonders of
your love
Restore to me The joy of your salvation. Restore to me, Restore to me!"

At that moment we both knew that was exactly what we needed from
our heavenly father, complete restoration.

I listened as he shared our story with our church family and then went on to sing the song, *"Restore to Me."* I bowed my head and listened to the instruments play and was able to thank God for this moment in my life. This moment where others could see how God can restore our lives if we only allow Him the chance.

I looked around the sanctuary at the people who had reached their hands out to us, loved us, cooked meals for us, prayed for us, and I watched the tears stream from their faces as they smiled.

The presence of the Lord was so strong this day and I was honored and proud to watch my husband share our story of grief, love, and triumph. I was in complete awe over the power of my Lord and Savior and His true amazing grace.

God can and will restore our hearts if we ask Him too. He can and will take the pain in our lives and turn it around to touch the lives of others. How amazing!

Father, thank you for this amazing moment. Thank you for using our story to touch the lives of so many. Use our story to bring glory to your name forever and ever. Amen.

~It is so hard to even imagine how and where life will go after you lose your child. The thought of God touching any lives through what we had been through was unimaginable to me. Through God's love and grace He can and will use your suffering to touch the lives of others. I will miss my daughter FOREVER. I will ache for her FOREVER. I will long to touch her FOREVER. Until then, I choose to let God use her NOW for His glory.

Day 31- True Peace

"But He was pierced for our transgressions, He was crushed for our iniquities; the punishment that brought us peace was upon Him, and by His wounds we are healed."

Isaiah 53:5

Happiness or sadness? Anxiety or Peace? Anger or Joy? Life happens, and as hard as we try we cannot always change the unforgettable and heartbreaking circumstances that life may, and probably will, throw our way.

Because of God we do have a choice on how we deal with those situations or how we allow Him to lead us through them. Peace is obtainable although many times it may seem like a million miles away, in fact its more than obtainable, it's possible!

In I Peter 5:7, Isaiah clearly tells all we need to do: "Cast all your anxiety on Him because He cares for you." Christ cares for us so much and can give us that peace and happiness we so deeply desire, even in the darkest moment of our life if we: a) fix our eyes on Jesus, and b) truly give our anxiety to Him! Give your fears, anxiety, and hopelessness to Him and allow Christ to heal your heart. Allow Christ to renew your heart and regain your Strength!

Today marks the one year anniversary since my sweet little Bethany Hope went to be with my Lord and Savior in Heaven. Although my selfish side longs for her to be here, I am at peace, true peace. My Savior continues to make me lean on Him and trust that He has a plan for my life and He will and has pulled me through every circumstance in my life, even when I remained uncertain.

Praise God He never gave up on me and never will. I long to be a servant, a witness, and a believer to myself, my family, and those Christ may put in my path.

I have learned that although time, along with Christ, can heal your heart, my heart will forever ache for my daughter. But Praise God He will always be there to get me through those moments where I need to let my heart miss her and let the tears flow. She is a part of my life now and until we are reunited with my Savior for eternity.

Father, Lead me into your arms now and forever. Allow me to choose peace and give you all of my anxiety. Thank you for caring for me that much and allow me to accept your love. Teach me to daily fix my eyes upon you and allow you to work in my life. Amen.

~Allowing yourself to come to a point where you can choose to be at peace with your child's death is a huge choice and accomplishment. Christ can and will bring you to this point if you allow Him to control you heart and you life. Who is in control of your heart today?

Day 32-It's all an Attitude!

"Work willingly at whatever you do, as though you were working for the Lord rather than for people. Remember that the Lord will give you an inheritance as your reward, and that the Master you are serving is Christ. "

Colossians 3:23-24

Like many moms I found myself trying to accomplish a hundred different tasks, as if I was the real life superwomen that every mom and wife tries to be. I had stayed up way too late finishing our shoeboxes for operation Christmas child.

If you are unaware of operation Christmas child, it is a wonderful program sponsored by Samaritan's purse. The concept is to fill a shoebox with gifts for either a boy or girl and then wrap it and drop it off at your local church or designated drop off area, and the boxes are then sent all over the world to children who would otherwise receive no gifts for Christmas.

I finished the boxes and hurried the kids off to bed, way too late! Early Sunday morning the alarm clock never had time to wake me up because my sweet husband squirming around ever so kindly woke me up way before I was ready.

Of all Sundays, he was singing in church and had to be there early to practice so, I was on my own and he was out the door. I laid with my head in the bed hoping the next five minutes of sleep I might get would feel like an hour, although my daughter was quick to swing open the door two minutes later shouting, "Daddy left, were going to be late!"

I unhappily jumped out of bed and the chaos began. Before my daughter could blink I had rollers in her hair and had practically morphed my five year old into his church clothes. My sweet eight year old son, who is not a morning person much like his mother, was for some reason quick to get ready this particular Sunday. I was not complaining! I quickly fed them all breakfast, as I begged them to not get their clothes dirty.

I somehow managed to get myself dressed in the mix of eating as I was getting dressed. We quickly jumped in the car and we were headed to church.

I breathed a sigh of relief as I looked at the clock and realized we were on time, YES, we made it! I pulled into the church parking Lot and just remembered, after all the hard work of packing those shoeboxes that I was supposed to bring to church, and they were still on the kitchen table.

I quickly turned the car around and snapped at the kids, "Why didn't you remind me to get the boxes"?

The children were having a special walk down of the boxes during the church service and I had forgotten them. As I was driving back home I could hear my children singing the praise and worship songs that were on the radio. I could feel God pulling at my heart. It was not my children's fault, it was my responsibility. Was it really that big of a deal if we were late to church?

The children that receive these boxes we made might not even be able to go to church and I am mad just because I'm late.

I realized that my attitude was all wrong.

I turned around and apologized to my kids and we all started joyfully singing to the Lord. I made it home, got the boxes, and returned to church with a better attitude. I returned with an attitude that I am blessed to have a church to go to even if I am a little late sometimes.

What's your attitude today and who are you taking that attitude out on? If we are doing a good deed with a sour attitude then are we really doing a good deed at all?

Remember to be grateful for the places you have to go and the people you have in your life. Our circumstances are not always the way we want them to be, but we can always go about each and every situation with the very best attitude possible.

Losing my daughter has taught me that I do not know what tomorrow may hold, so why would I waste today with a bad attitude and being angry at the ones Gods has blessed me to keep?

Today is vapor; our life with Christ is an Eternity! Don't waist that small vapor holding on to what we can't have. Use it to change the world around you with a simple smile and an attitude that reflects Christ in your life.

Father, forgive me for my selfish attitude and thank you for the children and the church you have given me. Help me to not get so wrapped up in the business of life that my attitude does not reflect one of gratefulness. Amen.

~Where is your attitude today, and who are you taking it out on? Life is and can seem uncontrollably busy at times, but it is not the end of the world if you are occasionally late. Remember to be thankful you have these places to go and a schedule to keep you busy in the first place. How is your attitude today, and what are you doing to start changing it for the better?

Day 33- Right or Wrong?

"But now, O Lord, You are our Father; we are the clay, and You are our potter; we are all the work of Your hand."

Isaiah 64:8

Imagine running into the middle of an intersection and having cars coming at you from every direction and you can't tell if the police man standing in the road is telling you to walk or stand still. You would feel lost, confused, frustrated? This seems to be my brain lately.

I feel as though I am standing in the intersection and cars are coming at me in every direction and I am screaming for them to stop and I just can't seem to understand what God is telling me to do. Am I supposed to walk or stop?

Where do I go from here?

Life seems so unpredictable, and yet everyone around me is continuing on with their next step as though they know exactly what to do.

Where is my answer?

Why do I still feel so lost some days? I'm a Christian right, God will take care of everything; the Sunday school answer, I know!

The truth is, my heart is aching so badly some days I wonder where God is. I think it is in those days that God really speaks to me. It is in those days that I realize God feels so far away because I have pushed Him so far away. How can I ask God to heal my heart when I fade away into the darkness of my grief and forbid myself to even crack a smile?

If I push God away, I am the one not letting Him work in my life. I realized I was scared to let God heal my heart. If God heals my heart and I smile again, then that means I don't hurt over my daughter anymore. If

I laugh with my children, then I'm not mourning my daughter's death, or at least that's how I thought it would seem.

There is no right or wrong, but I do know it's ok to feel, and it is ok to allow God to let you smile and feel joy in your life again, in fact it's healing! I will always miss her, and she will always be part of my life.

I am learning to smile when I think about her, and to smile when I glance at her picture hanging in my house. My memories of her can be because of the joy God has brought back into my life and not only of the sadness of her death. I will praise her life because she was fearfully and wonderfully made. I will love her and honor her life because she is a miracle. Someone on a forum once told me that they imagined an angel coming down and carrying their child straight into the arms of Jesus. I loved this because it took a moment that I remember as heartbreaking and turned it into something beautiful.

Father, Some days I'm not sure I can distinguish what's right and what's wrong, but Lord I know you are right in my life. Lord, show me your direction and show me that it's ok to feel and it's ok to be happy or sad. Allow me to feel your love today. Amen.

~Knowing what's right or wrong in this journey can sometimes make anyone's head spin out of control. There is no right or wrong answer to what your heart is feeling. It is ok to laugh, cry, scream or even let loose and run wild around house; if of course that is what you need to do! The point is; you decide how you feel and what you are willing to do with those feelings. Take the memories you have of your child and learn to find joy in them. Miss your child and cry on the days you need to just let out the pain. Find what works for you.

_____
_____
_____
_____
_____
_____
_____
_____
_____
_____
_____
_____
_____
_____
_____
_____
_____
_____
_____
_____
_____
_____
_____
_____
_____
_____
_____
_____
_____
_____
_____
_____
_____

Day 34-JOY

"I prayed to the LORD, and He answered me. He freed me from all my fears. Those who look to Him for help will be radiant with joy; no shadow of shame will darken their faces. In my desperation I prayed, and the LORD listened; He saved me from all my troubles. For the angel of the LORD is a guard; He surrounds and defends all who fear Him." Psalm 34:4-7

I was driving to the grocery store this morning enjoying the simple peace and quiet I found surrounding me this day. I was listening to one of my favorite Christian radio stations as they were talking.

They were challenging their listeners to sum up their life in one word, one word that would describe the last year of your life. Without even thinking the word joy came to my mind, which then struck me as odd, considering the details of the last year of my life.

This had been the hardest year of my life and, to many, would be considered the worst year; yet, I believe this was the best year of my life! How on earth can I sit here and say that the year my daughter died and I suffered extreme medical problems was the best year of my life?

It's simple, really it is: Joy.

Joy in my Lord and Savior, Jesus Christ. I was lost this year as I struggled through day after day on this new journey and yet my Savior was there day after day after day, leading, guiding, providing, and showing me that joy can triumph grief.

He has shown me joy in my marriage, my children, mended family relationships, and the joy of watching my seven year old son accept Christ as His Savior. In the midst of darkness my only hope was to fall into the arms of my Savior and pray He would not only catch me, but pick me back up again, and not only did He pick up time after time, He brought joy into my life when I never thought I would smile again.

I now aim to allow Christ to show me joy no matter what situation may come my way. He will never leave me and He will always be there willing and ready to show me joy and hope for a new day.

What's your word of the year?

Will you commit to letting Jesus Christ show you joy even in the darkest moments of your life? God never promised that our life would be easy, but He did promise to never leave our side! Are you ready to cling to that promise and allow Christ to lead your heart today and forevermore?

Father, thank you for the joy you have brought back into my life. Thank you for teaching me that you will never leave my side and you will continue you to pick me up every time I need you. Allow me to commit this joy into my life from now until forevermore, Amen!

~Let your heart be free. Let go of whatever is still holding you back and finally give it all to Jesus. He is waiting with open arms to love you and protect you from here until forever, just open your heart and let Him in. What is your word for the year and how do you choose to live your life from here on out?

_____

_____

_____

_____

_____

_____

_____

_____

_____

_____

_____

_____

_____

_____

_____

_____

_____

_____

_____

_____

_____

_____

_____

_____

_____

_____

_____

_____

_____

_____

_____

_____

For You created my inmost being;
You knit me together in my mother's womb.
Psalms 139:13

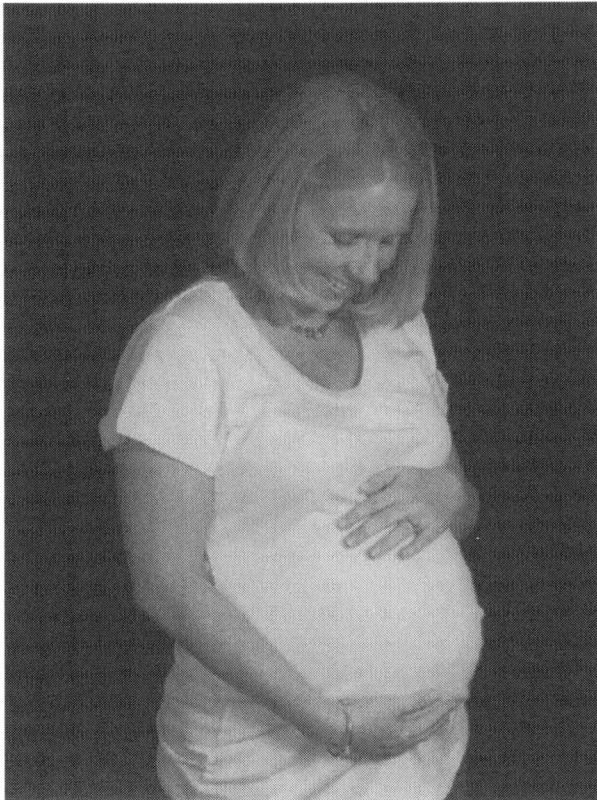

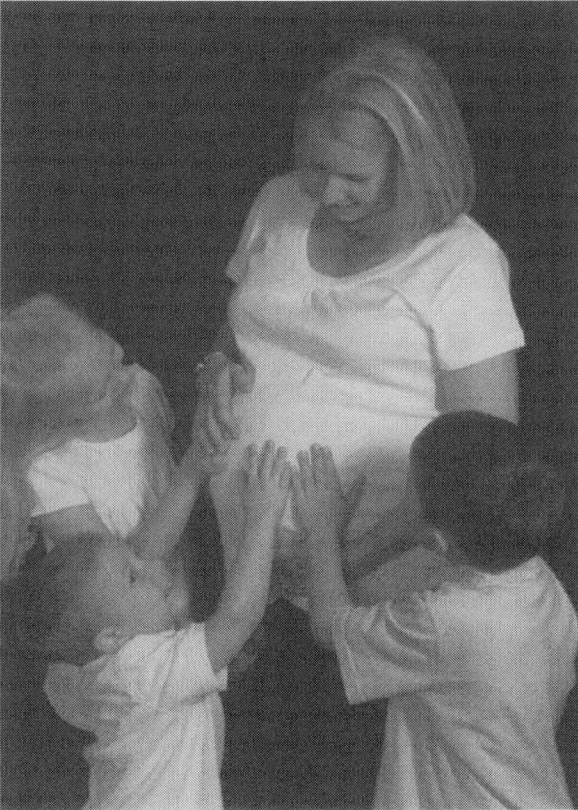

"I Will Praise You in This Storm" By: Casting Crowns
I was sure by now
God You would have reached down
And wiped our tears away
Stepped in and saved the day
But once again, I say "Amen", and it's still raining
As the thunder rolls
I barely hear Your whisper through the rain
"I'm with you"
And as Your mercy falls
I raise my hands and praise the God who gives
And takes away

And I'll praise You in this storm And I will lift my hands
For You are who You are No matter where I am
And every tear I've cried You hold in Your hand
You never left my side And though my heart is torn
I will praise You in this storm

I remember when I stumbled in the wind
You heard my cry to you And you raised me up again
My strength is almost gone How can I carry on
If I can't find You
But as the thunder rolls
I barely hear You whisper through the rain
"I'm with you"
And as Your mercy falls
I raise my hands and praise the God who gives
And takes away

And I'll praise You in this storm
And I will lift my hands For You are who You are
No matter where I am And every tear I've cried
You hold in Your hand You never left my side
And though my heart is torn I will praise You in this storm

I lift my eyes unto the hills Where does my help come from?
My help comes from the Lord The Maker of Heaven and Earth.

Finding Jesus Christ

"For God so loved the world that He gave His one and only Son, that whoever believes in Him shall not perish but have eternal life". John 3:16

"If you confess with your mouth the Lord Jesus and believe in your heart that God has raised Him from the dead, you will be saved. For with the heart one believes to righteousness, and with the mouth confession is made to salvation". Romans 10:9

If you have read my story and want to have the same joy I have even in the darkest moment of your life, I encourage you to find Jesus. God sent His only son Jesus to die on a cross so that you and I could have eternal life. To ask Jesus Christ into your heart you must acknowledge in your heart that Jesus is the Son of God. Confess with your mouth that He is the son of God. Believe that Jesus died on a cross to save you from your sins, and was raised from the dead three days later. Repent of your sins and be baptized.

Prayer of Salvation:

"God, I admit that I am a sinner, and I have not lived my life for you. I believe that Jesus is your son and died on a cross to save me from my sins. Please forgive me for my sins and come into my heart as my Lord and Savior. I love you Lord Jesus. Amen".

Getting Plugged In:

If you have prayed this prayer of salvation, then I encourage you to find a church in your area to be baptized in. Getting plugged into a church will allow you to grow in your relationship with Christ. Remember, sometimes it takes time to find a church that fits your needs just right. Don't be discouraged if you visit a church and you do not feel like it is right for you. Please visit others until you find exactly where God wants you to be.

To contact me:

Blog- http://www.myangelwithgod.blogspot.com/

E-mail- stillinmyarms@gmail.com

Thank you to my dear friend, Valerie Crawford, for your sacrifice and time in proofreading this book.

Resources

These are a list of resources available to guide you through this difficult time.

- National Stillbirth Society- http://www.stillnomore.org/
- Sufficient Grace Ministries- A great place dedicated to helping parents after a loss. They will make a memory book of your child at no cost to the parents. http://www.sufficientgrace.net/
- A forum dedicated to talking about the loss of a child. http://stillbirthforum.com/forum/
- Now I Lay Me Down To Sleep is a group of photographers who capture pictures of your lost child at no cost to the parents. http://www.nowilaymedowntosleep.org/
- This is the blog of Angie Smith. She is a godly women who has inspired hundreds of women to follow Christ after her daughter went to be with Jesus: http://audreycaroline.blogspot.com/

Made in the USA
Columbia, SC
03 December 2019